The Beauty Experiment

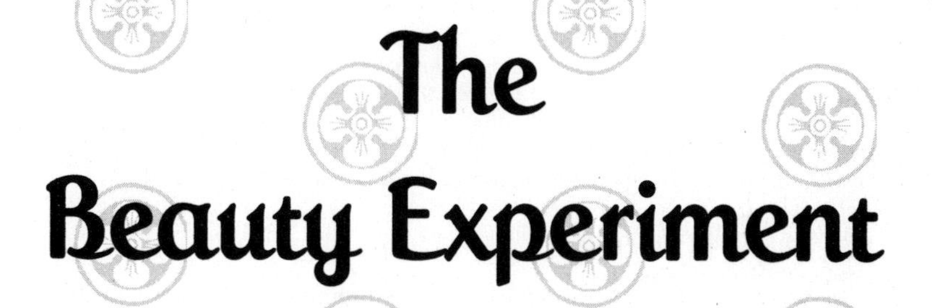

The Beauty Experiment

How I Skipped Lipstick,
Ditched Fashion,
Faced the World Without Concealer
. . . and Learned to Love the Real Me

PHOEBE BAKER HYDE

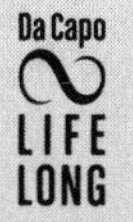

DA CAPO LIFELONG
A MEMBER OF THE PERSEUS BOOKS GROUP

Some individuals' names and identifying details have been changed, and in Chapter 6 two interactions have been combined.

Printed in the United States of America. For information, address Da Capo Press, 44 Farnsworth Street, 3rd Floor, Boston, MA 02210.

Designed by Linda Mark
Set in 11 point Photina Std by the Perseus Books Group

Library of Congress Cataloging-in-Publication Data
Hyde, Phoebe Baker.
The beauty experiment : how I skipped lipstick, ditched fashion, faced the world without concealer . . . and learned to love the real me / Phoebe Baker Hyde.—1st Da Capo Press ed.
p. cm.
Includes bibliographical references and index.
ISBN 978-0-7382-1465-8 (pbk. : alk. paper)—ISBN 978-0-7382-1543-3 (e-book)
1. Beauty, Personal—Psychological aspects. 2. Self-esteem in women. 3. Self-acceptance in women. 4. Self-perception in women. 5. Clothing and dress—Psychological aspects. I. Title.
HQ1219.H93 2013
111'.85—dc23

2012035590

First Da Capo Press edition 2013
Published by Da Capo Press
A Member of the Perseus Books Group
www.dacapopress.com

10 9 8 7 6 5 4 3 2 1

For Harriet Maeyu and Molly Maddox,
and for every woman who knows her inner voice

Contents

INTRODUCTION ix

1 THE RED DRESS 1

2 THE BEAUTY EXPERIMENT 23

3 THE HAIR QUESTIONS 33

4 TWO HALF-MOONS OF PEACH PASTE 49

5 THE DAY I COVERED THE MIRRORS 65

6 ITSY BITSY TEENY-WEENY FERTILITY ADVERTISEMENT 87

7 THE PROFESSIONALS 105

8 PRETTY MIND 123

9 A LANGUAGE EVERY BODY SPEAKS 137

10 THE EMPTY JAR 163

11 Outgrowing the Gown 183

12 Burn Like the Sun at Midday 203

About the Survey 219

Notes 221

Readings 229

Acknowledgments 231

Introduction

THIS IS WHO I AM: A WOMAN. I'm a daughter, a sister, a friend, a wife, and a mother. At age seven, I was a girl with braids and rainbow hair clips, and at thirteen, I became a teenager with acne, orthodontics, and teased bangs. At nineteen, I was a college student battling her freshman twenty-five, then a new graduate with a discount poly-blend office wardrobe. For nearly a decade after that, I was an independent young woman in confusing relationships who paired thrift-store finds with designer shoes. At twenty-eight, I became an overjoyed fiancée with a shiny new ring, then an anxious newlywed with a new mortgage. When I was thirty-one, I swelled up into a pregnant goddess with superlative melons, then collapsed, nine months later, into a zombie with magenta undereye bags. Then that happened again. Today, at thirty-seven, I am a busy work-at-home parent and spouse. On most days, I wear jeans, and shoes with traction. I have a yoga membership I probably won't use up. On Fridays, I drink a beer in front of the television and fall asleep before ten.

Despite this remarkably average female chronology, I feel I have one small, hard-won feature that is extraordinary. It is this: When I look in the mirror, I don't see wrinkles, anxiety, zits, or exhaustion, although they are all there. Instead, I see a face, a person, a personality, a life. If someone asked me if I felt beautiful, I would have to answer honestly: yes.

I didn't start out this way. Some might call me "low maintenance," but in the three-and-a-half decades of my life, I've done hundreds of ridiculous, bizarre, and embarrassing things in beauty's name. I constipated myself with chocolate diet shakes the summer I was fifteen. I broke in a pair of punishingly uncomfortable high heels by wearing them with hiking socks and jogging laps around a parking lot. I was caught kickboxing in my room wearing three sweaters and a raincoat in hopes of dropping weight before a college formal. Convinced of the powers of exfoliation, I tried to scrub the cystic acne off my back with a foot pumice. I once paid a great deal of money for a bikini wax that left me polka-dotted with blood from the crotch down, and another time, I mutely obeyed a teenage beauty technician who barked "Lie still" while caustic eyelash-dying solution burned under my lids. I felt perversely thrilled, afterward, that the treatment had only fogged my peripheral vision. I had not actually gone blind.

In college, I was an anthropology major, trained to recognize ritualistic, illogical, and masochistic behaviors in other cultures. But when it came to my own beauty craziness, and the insistent voice in my head that drove me to it, I simply didn't care to question. This crap seemed trivial, and I had so many other, better, things to think about: my professional aspirations, my love life, and the world around me. Sure, my own lack of physical beauty and constant need for personal correction and enhancement were often foremost in my mind—usually when I wished they weren't—but I assumed that one day I'd simply outgrow the freaky diets, the wardrobe crises, and the occasional substitution of prettiness for poise. For thirty-two years, I lived with the enigma of my female beauty craziness the way I lived with the Bermuda Triangle: it was weird and creepy in its persistence, but not my problem to solve.

Things changed in late 2005—or began changing then. I was living in San Francisco with my husband, John, my best friend and the great love of my life, when he was transferred to Hong Kong by his company. This was something we'd both long been hoping for: John is a Chinese American who was born in Taiwan, and this move would give him a chance to reconnect with the Chinese culture and language as an adult. As an avid overseas traveler, I was thrilled to be going abroad for more than a few weeks. We'd been in San Francisco only a few months—I had yet to establish a professional or social network and figured I could make the classic artist's bargain anywhere in the world: taking a low-profile day job in exchange for the luxury of time to write. What Hong Kong might offer in terms of day jobs was less clear, but in the weeks before the move, I fixated on another joyful development: I'd just become pregnant with our first child. John worried about having our baby so far from family, but I brushed these concerns off. This was adventure! This was life!

Our flight to Hong Kong was my first business-class seat ever, and we were met the day after our arrival by a team of relocation specialists—both Chinese and European—in silk scarves, bejeweled shoes, blowouts, and Chanel suits. (They might have been knockoff Chanel suits—but how would I have known? Forty-eight hours earlier, I'd been munching spirulina bars from the Rainbow grocery and selling engineered socks to female triathletes in Noe Valley.) These relocation specialists came with advice for a wide-eyed and inexperienced expatriate, and I listened up. At their recommendations, we picked a private hospital and a safe, convenient address (with a pool!), and I joined a women's club. I went to some club events and started making lunch dates. Hong Kong, like many other cosmopolitan cities outside America, is a place where street shoes vastly outnumber sneakers, and since it seemed the thing to do, I started dressing up for those lunch dates. I began wearing foundation to the grocery store and drifting into shops to sample hundred-dollar cosmetics. When I went to the hospital to have our baby, I took mascara along for those all-important first pictures and postpartum visits—all from people I'd known only a few months.

When the baby weight didn't come off as fast as online forums promised, I tried to counteract my hideous rib-cage spreading by wearing a spandex corset five hours a day. I bought thicker makeup and brighter lipstick to disguise the haggard face I met in the mirror. Weekly, sometimes daily, I found myself digging through bins at a street-side sample warehouse near our apartment, believing something at the bottom of the bin would have the power to make me happy, or satisfied, or sexy, or whatever it was that suddenly, inexplicably, I wasn't.

In February 2007, I threw up the white flag of surrender. I had become a nervous, critical, angry, insecure woman. I was not the woman or the role model I wanted to be, especially in front of a big-eyed baby daughter. I was at war with the world around me and at war with myself—the only self I had. And so I swore off Beauty and all her trappings: makeup, new clothes, salon haircuts, jewelry, the works. I told very few people what I was doing, took detailed but sporadic notes, and had only a vague sense of a goal: something needed to change for the better.

Technically, my beauty experiment lasted for a little more than a year. It was a strange, uncomfortable thirteen months, and while I'd like to report that it magically cured me of beauty craziness, it did not. What happened was more like what happens when you stare at those poster-size optical illusions, the ones that look like a chaos of computer-generated black dots—at first. If you look at the dots long enough, though, unfocusing your eyes and relaxing your brain, a scene emerges in the chaos. A happy dolphin swims through a hoop; fish flicker behind stalks of kelp. The picture becomes startlingly clear, and you can't believe you ever missed it. It was these kinds of shapes and patterns I noticed during the year of my experiment. They were often surprising, sometimes confusing, and usually didn't reflect well on me. Some were so elemental they seemed impossible to change. The woman I was at the end of my beauty experiment differed from the woman who started it, but I was still making journal entries filled with questions, not answers.

Luckily, I didn't write this book then. I was too busy with an international move back to the United States, an active toddler, and a second pregnancy. Out of necessity, I pushed my beauty experiment and its disheartening—and seemingly inconclusive—results aside. My life changed and changed again. My rib cage spread another inch, and my baby daughter transformed herself from an infant repository of motherly angst into a real kid confronting the world of shopping malls and miniature plastic-glitter high heels. I made new friends in the United States and began having new, but often familiar, conversations about beauty—losing it, seeking it, buying it, trying to find it beyond the parameters of a good figure and pretty face. I realized that beauty craziness was not a problem to be solved, but a lens through which I could read—and better understand—many aspects of female experience.

I returned to my experiment then, rereading the observations in my notes and reexamining the feelings I had during that strange year. I began to think more critically and more generously about the lives of women I knew. I gathered facts about the beauty industries and read up on women's history and the real challenges facing all of us—women, men, families, parents, daughters and sons, caregivers and breadwinners—as we negotiate a world where culture, gender, and economic identities are as jumbled up as junk in a messy purse.

One morning I happened across *Newsweek*'s online "Beauty Breakdown" interactive feature, an estimate of what female "divas" in every age range spend on beauty in a year. The numbers seemed grossly exaggerated to me, and not representative of any real woman I'd ever met. At the same time, those supersized diva silhouettes were very familiar—public phantoms of femaleness against which I was invited to measure my femininity and, more often than not, come up short.* In response, I designed and posted the "Beauty Experiment Surveys" online—a forty-four-question investigation of women's beauty habits and experiences, as well as a shorter survey for men.

This book encompasses all these elements: my surveys' chorus of more than five hundred anonymous voices, the conversational insights of acquaintances and friends, the measured wisdom of female writers and researchers, and even the silent presence of women only tangentially impacted by American and European standards of femininity, but affected all the same.

Primarily, though, this is the story of two women, both of them me.

---

*As of February 2012, the feature was still accessible at http://www.thedailybeast.com/newsweek/features/2010/the-beauty-breakdown.html.

Imagine a set of makeover shots. The first shots—the numbered chapters in this book—show "before and during" as I secretly embarked on my experiment in Hong Kong. The second shots—the snapshots at the ends of chapters—are the "after" shots, me still becoming myself in the years since the experiment concluded. I don't look drastically different—same face, same body, same wardrobe, more or less, just a few years further into life. But these snapshots reveal a woman a little less afraid of looking wrong, a little more assured of her appeal, and a lot quicker to laugh at her mistakes. Nearly five years since the day she tossed her makeup, this is a woman who finally knows how to respond with wisdom and compassion to the voice of beauty craziness in her head.

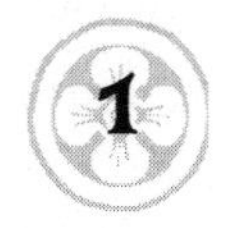

The Red Dress

No, it was not *right* . . . for oh these men, these women, were all thinking—"What's Mabel wearing? What a fright she looks!"

—Mabel Waring in *The New Dress*,
by Victorian author Virginia Woolf

Hong Kong, February 2007

The crimson party invitation was stuck in the dining-room mirror like a *hong bao*—one of the fat, tantalizing red envelopes of cash that children get on the Chinese New Year. John had brought it home from the office a few days ago and tucked it in the frame; since then my eyes had flicked to it repeatedly while spooning pabulum into Hattie's mouth. In Hong Kong the season of winter holidays extended into February, the end of the lunar year, when John's firm held its company-wide Chinese New Year gala. Last year's party had been so big it was held in the Hong Kong Convention Center. With entertainment by a

Cantopop star and trapeze artist during the cocktail hour, it had lived up to its theme: *Glitz*. This year's party theme was printed on the invitation in glittering flames: *Red-Hot!* The implication was blisteringly clear: I needed a hot new dress—a *red* one.

It was important that I look great, I thought, plucking the invite out of the mirror for the eighth or ninth time and fingering it. There were many reasons. The shallowest of these was that this year we might be seated with the firm's partners. Last year, when we were newbies on the island, there had been some question as to whether I was of automatic *Glitz*-inclusion status: Important Person's Attendant Wife. In the end I'd made the cut and had worn a dress from the back of my closet—a slim, black, bias-cut thrift-store score that had squeezed a five-months-pregnant bump prettily. In a perverse *let's see,* I'd recently tried it on. No go. Of motherhood's aftermath, it forgave zero.

Another reason I felt I deserved a new dress was that Hattie's birth had been a nasty blur of fear, gas masks, and screaming in Cantonese. Then, while John and I were finally dialing our families with the good news, a nearsighted obstetrician apologized for missing a significant heart defect on every one of the prenatal scans. That was why all the screaming, all the panic, all the vacuuming in delivery, he explained. Our daughter had a ventricular septal defect of middle size: something to get tested, something to watch.

The resulting fear and confusion then stretched across weeks and international boundaries as John returned to a busy work and travel schedule and I was left carting a newborn who might or might not need heart surgery to the pediatricians and cardiologists.* To this hardship I could add the

* She did not need it or get it, and so far she is completely fine.

distance and time difference between Hong Kong and the United States, the challenge of breast-feeding in a class-conscious country averse to the idea unless you are a pig farmer's wife, ten months of sleep in four-hour intervals, wearing the goddamned spandex girdle, and thousands of before-bed crunches. I wasn't the math whiz in the family, but when I summed it all up, it equaled the splurge of a new party dress with change to spare.

"I want you to see me looking beautiful," I said to John when he was hunched over his dinner late that night. As our sole breadwinner now, he would have to pay for the outfit. "But I won't go overboard. You know that."

"I know," he said, and he looked up with the sweetly haggard expression he'd worn since Hattie's birth. It was the face of trying for excellence when you barely had the energy for good.

During his paternity leave, John had cooked us home-style Chinese meals every day. He had taken hundreds of pictures of Hattie, and when she wailed, he played her the Bach Variations on his cello. We were a family. But then those two happy weeks ended. In his new position as an accounting ninja, John was responsible for building a specialty branch of the firm's business, a mandate that lay in direct conflict with the demands of budding family life. There was little he could do for Hattie and me when he came home at 11:00 p.m., or from his hotel room in Seoul, except work harder and more diligently so that he'd become indispensable.

One of the things that usually made me feel close to John—apart from our shared love of the arts—was his habit of complete intellectual absorption that mirrored and often outpaced my own. I understood how days and cities and even one's own body could fall away when the mind was in the sway of a difficult problem or intriguing idea. In the earlier days of our relationship, a kiss, the chorus of a good song, or even a dangled takeout menu could break the spell. Recently, I despaired of ever getting the man to look up from his laptop. I hoped the saying about red sports cars getting into more trouble held true for red party dresses, too.

WHEN YOU WAKE UP EARLY IN HONG KONG AND OPEN A WINDOW, the fecund, slightly tangy odor wafting in is the smell of the sale. Hong Kong is one of the world's great shopping capitals, not only because so much merchandise is produced there, but because retail, especially garment retail, pervades every possible urban crevice and rural alley. You can browse in a boutique while a phalanx of saleswomen ply you with oolong tea, or you can haggle with a one-armed, gold-toothed vendor in a seaside market. You can order a one-of-a-kind crocodile-skin handbag with your monogram inlaid in gold. Or, you can ascend to the fifth floor of a condemned building, give the secret knock, and watch the walls slide back to reveal the epicenter of the faux–designer handbag universe, replete with hundreds of one-of-a-kind pieces made in the very same factories, with the very same materials, possibly using the very same crocodiles. An army of tailors can make you a bespoke suit overnight, and miles of street-level stalls offer samples and couture knockoffs right next to chandeliered, marble-floored retail palaces. They are malls, but it's hard to call them that.

It would have made sense, in this environment, to be strategic about a big purchase, taking my time and assessing my options. But the more I thought about how deeply I deserved the red dress, how luxurious it would make me feel, and how splendid it would make me look, the more I anticipated and delayed. In the end I gave myself only one afternoon to shop: five hours to locate the needle of red-hot perfection in Hong Kong's retail haystack—all while attending to a sticky-fingered infant in a stroller.

I chose Pacific Place, a shopping center not dripping with Gucci and Dior but one that was still anchored by upscale department stores. In these bigger stores the saleswomen would advance three or four at a time to help and smile, and most of them spoke retail English. But Pacific Place was also adjacent to some of Hong Kong's raised pedestrian walkways, along which were tens of smaller, cheaper local boutiques staffed by Cantonese speakers who would leave me alone to try things on. I'd start there.

It had been too long since I'd been dress shopping. I'd thought I could negotiate with some of the Chinese-made clothes, but they bit into my rib cage, pinched me under the armpits, and refused to close over my backside and hips.* The sizing was unfathomable, too. Was a 210 equivalent to an American 8? A British 14? My waist measurement? No idea. Bust? Mine was too large, that was clear.

Porn queen, said my familiar inner Voice when I tried on a plunging blazer-gone-wrong style. I switched to a short, shapeless baby-doll confection, but that was no good either. *Old Mother Hubbard gets run over by the lacemobile!*

Decisively, I changed tack. Spinning Hattie's stroller on one wheel, I abandoned the tiny shops reeking of polyester and acetate and headed into Pacific Place to try Seibu, a big Japanese department store. Many of the racks had been denuded by shoppers attending earlier holiday parties, so the fanciest

* The average Chinese female is five foot four, weighs 125 pounds, and has bust-waist-hip measurements of 31-28-35. The average American female is five foot four, weighs 155 pounds, and measures 37-34-42.

stuff was gone, but now I was hunting for the "simple wrap dress" my upstairs neighbor and friend Anne had counseled.

Anne was a Brit guided by excellent taste and a strict adherence to practical economy. "A wrap dress will be more useful than some frilly party frock," she'd advised. "And it can still look quite nice." I did see how sensible this was, so I dumped a few wrap dresses over the hood of the stroller and tried again. As I'd suspected, that style was too plunging for my height, too clingy for my rear, and just too plain for my ambitions. *Red-Hot* was the theme, and red-hot I must be.

I was slumped on the cold dressing-room bench, wallowing, when Hattie Mae woke up from her stroller nap. As a barometer of the maternal climate, she was rapid and precise. She saw the pained grimace on my face, matched it, and, because she'd been securely belted in for upward of two hours, started to cry and buck. "I know, baby, I know," I said flinging the wraps aside and driving the stroller out of the department store at a run.

Had I been back home, in the States, I would have headed straight for Marshall's, Filene's Basement, or Century 21: name-brand quality, reasonable prices. As a last resort, I would have called a friend, who could have loaned me a red dress or otherwise put a stop to this madness with a better idea: wear red shoes, wear a red scarf, wear red lipstick. Here, though, the alternative to upscale stores was limited to the dusty bins in roadside stalls, and the pool of close friends I could have borrowed from was limited to Anne, who had five inches on me.

But Hong Kong did offer something unique to someone like me. I slowed us to a walk as I thought of it, fishing an overpriced, imported baby snack out of my bag and dropping it in Hattie's lap. Having been marked off as "dependent housewife" on the HK government form and having arrived with no work visa, no local friends, no professional community, no relatives to hand the baby off to for ten minutes, and no Cantonese, it often felt as if I were floating in a bubble through Hong Kong's super-air-conditioned cafés and malls. It was not a bubble of snobbery but one of separateness, my expatriate status being one of disengagement, isolation, and triviality. Against this social chill I'd discovered there were two measures I could take. First, I could surround myself with other expatriate women, and had. Second, draped over Hong Kong's rattan chairs like a forgotten cashmere shawl was a warm, comforting sense of Occidental wealth and privilege left over from the city's colonial days. When we arrived I hadn't thought I'd ever want or need it, but today it seemed quite easy—and right—to put on.

At the end of the atrium, I spotted a Vivienne Tam boutique, ablaze with end-of-season markdowns and carpeted with infant-friendly orange plush. The Voice in my head—the one that had just made wiseass cracks about those terrible, cheap dresses—now murmured in earnest, *Just go in there and buy something. This is how it's done.*

I threw my shoulders back and ran my fingers through my disheveled white-girl hair, and we went in. Banking on the boredom of the saleswomen, I unbuckled Hattie and set her down to crawl around on the thick carpet. In this store there were tens of marvelous dresses. Many of them fit my American frame. Some even looked good. The best one was a short velvet dress with a wide satin sash that neither revealed nor pinched. Unfortunately, it was black.

"We do have that one in another color," said an intuitive saleswoman, catching the scent of hopefulness wafting off me as I stood before the mirror. "In red." She pointed at the window. "I can take it off the mannequin for you."

"No, no," I said, but looked over. My pulse quickened with a surge of consumerist destiny.

That's the one.

"All right, maybe," I croaked. "Yes, I'd like to try it on."

The skirt was short. The sleeves were billowy and long, with a row of covered buttons at each cuff. The waistline was forgiving—elastic!—but covered with the satin ribbon. And the red velvet fabric, while a shade too bluish for my complexion, was blissfully soft, the kind of texture I liked to swaddle Hattie in but didn't squander on my own chapped skin. The dress had a boatneck, too, so my milk-inflated chest would be covered by a pattern of sheer cutouts in the velvet. It was demure but dramatic. I would be a red-hot phoenix rising from the ashes of new motherhood. I would be beautiful.

I bought it quickly, before I could change my mind or let the price settle in. One saleslady distracted me with questions about Hattie's ancestry, while the other rang up the sale.

"*Shi,*" I answered one of the salesladies, slipping the credit card across the counter, "*ta baba shi Zhongwen*" (Yes, her father is Chinese).

"Have your maid steam the wrinkles out before the party," the elder one told me knowingly as she carefully wrapped the dress in tissue and laid it gently in an oversize red shopping bag.

I nodded as if I had one.

Ordinarily, I rode the 25M bus home from Pacific Place, clamping our stroller between my knees and clinging desperately to a strap as the giant double-decker farted uphill. Today, however, I took an elevator up to the lobby of the Shangri La hotel. There, the bellman hailed me a cab and held my precious dress while I settled Hattie in the seat. As our taxi glided into traffic, I realized the only other dress I'd ever spent so much on was my wedding dress, and that was not much more.

I leaned back in the taxi, dizzy and warm, feeling that I'd had my way with the world. This dress was cake for breakfast, a martini before noon.

ঌ

FOR SEVERAL DAYS, THE DRESS HUNG IN MY CLOSET, CONCEALED BY its neighbors. I did not get the fantasy out and try it on; familiarity might have ruined the delight. Instead, I was filled with secret satisfaction, like a child with candy hidden under her pillow, or an investment banker with a certain offshore account. The point was not in using it but in having it.

Late one weeknight I finally told John about the dress. I knew I needed to manage the information carefully, because in addition to being an accountant's accountant, John is a man who pays with exact change, who once drove seven miles to return a bag of spoiled green beans, and who had questioned the necessity of crib-size sheets. Couldn't we just take the crib mattress out and wrap regular sheets around it? (I could, and did for a long while, until I covertly shelled out the sixteen bucks.)

"So, I bought a dress for the party," I said quietly. "Hattie and I went down to Pacific Place. It's pretty fancy. It's *de-sign-er.*"

John grimaced uncomfortably, probably wishing we'd discussed parameters when he'd agreed to the purchase.

"Guess how much I paid," I asked him.

He was tired, his mental-calculator TV addled. "A thousand dollars," he guessed miserably.

"No way!" I cried. "Much less than that! End-of-season markdown!" I beamed like Bob Barker as I revealed the actual price, a steal. Now we were both relieved. Now we were both excited and happy about the dress.

The morning of the party, I took the red velvet dress out, put it on, and walked into the main room to model it. Hattie was deeply involved with a collapsible vegetable steamer, and John was reading a work document.

"John. Johnny."

It took him a few moments to refocus his consciousness. Blinking, he took in the color, sleeves, and cutouts at the neck.

"It's . . . nice," he said finally, the strain of finding words obvious on his face.

"You don't like it?"

"It's just—different from what I expected," he said. "You usually like to show . . . " He gestured to his chest and arms.

"Well, this is much more elegant," I said. "I don't know if dresses like that . . . are really appropriate anymore. Low-cut, or supertight, or with an open back or something. I don't look the way I used to."

John gazed wistfully at the silent, solvable problems in his accounting literature and then dutifully laid it aside. "I think you should wear whatever you want," he said.

My eyes stung. Our apartment had mirrors in the main room, and I shoved the dining chairs aside so I could look at myself in one. Why was I not feeling the delight I'd felt in the shop? In the shop, the salesladies had crooned and twittered!

"It doesn't look exactly right with my hair in a ponytail and bare feet," I protested, poofing and smoothing the dress, trying to coax its showroom beauty from it. "Obviously, I should have bare legs with a dress like this, but Hong Kong people don't do bare legs in February. Even though it's warmer than LA, where people never wear stockings, ever. I was thinking black stockings, but they just seem way too dark for this red."

"I think black would be okay," John said.

"No! I need nude or champagne." I began smacking wrinkles out of the uncooperative dress. "I have no idea what shoes I'm going to wear with it, either. All I have are those funeral shoes and a bunch of pregnant-lady shoes. This kind of dress is supposed to have black pumps. Patent." I glared at myself in the mirror, furious now with the dress, and its betrayal. "And how," I cried out, desperate, "are black pumps going to magically fucking appear by five o'clock?"

I collapsed into the couch, the velvet Juliet sleeves flinging wide. This behavior was very, very bad, and I knew it, but I was as committed to the role as I was disgusted by it.

"Look," John said, his own tone desperate, his heart overtaxed by female intangibles. "Let's all go eat lunch somewhere, and then we can get you some shoes and stockings. Okay?"

"Really?"

"Yes. It's a nice dress. You're going to look great in it."

I was only partially convinced.

We went out and bought me some shoes, and a few hours later we got ready for the party. I shaved and shampooed and conditioned in the shower for nearly forty minutes; I put my hair in an updo, then took the whole thing out; I experimented with different lipsticks and eyeliners and shimmied into the dress at the end, tying and retying the silk belt until I'd achieved a perfect bow of medium size, the ends of the ribbon hanging with asymmetrical casualness a half-inch apart. When I got into the taxi, wrapped up tight in my dress coat with new black patent-leather peep-toe pumps sparkling on my feet, I felt as beautiful and captivating as the glitter of Hong Kong at night. But when we got out and I unbuttoned my coat, I noticed that the wide ribbon belt had folded in half in the taxi. It no longer lay flat over the elastic waist. This problem consumed me as we rode the escalator up into the party. I tried to flatten the crease by reversing the fold.

"What are you doing?" John asked as I poked his ribs with my elbow. "It looks fine. Leave it alone."

I did not. I kept one hand on my waist as John and I wandered into the cocktail hour and got drinks.

No matter how many times I walked into a mostly Asian crowd on John's arm, I still heard what I believed to be a murmur of unpleasant surprise. In my mind I translated it as, "Why *her* when a successful guy like him could have a thinner, prettier Asian wife?" John chatted and laughed with some of his colleagues as I stood stiffly by his side. One of them was a native of Hong Kong who'd studied in Canada. Her open-necked dress showed off white, delicate collarbones, a tiny rib cage, and slender arms. The black silk was glossy, trim and elegant in the dim lighting. In the five minutes I stood beside her, my dramatic red dress soured and went bad. My look had more in common with the administrative assistants giggling around the photo pavilion. There were beads and sequins in their updos, and some wore floor-length satin gowns. They seemed to be having the fun that I'd imagined for myself.

The dinner seating was more relaxed than I had anticipated, which was now a relief. I'd been looking forward all week to some adult conversation, but had zip to contribute to a heated conversation about US GAAP,* so I turned to the wine for help. After a glass or two, the velvet began to feel nice again against my skin, and I ignored the accounting shoptalk and focused on the deliciousness of a meal that was not cold, leftover scrambled eggs and teething biscuits. But as the dress had betrayed me, so did my liquid burgundy friend. I went out to

* US GAAP: United States Generally Accepted Accounting Principles.

the restroom, teetering, intent on not falling down in the new shoes—and when I got back I found John posed for a photo with the fashionable colleague and a few others. Awkwardly, I skipped over to him—ruining the shot—and sat down possessively in his lap.

"Hey, you're blocking everyone," John objected, adjusting my position. There was laughter with an undercurrent of grumbling as everyone made room for me. The picture was taken again with me in it—a smear of red against a field of black.

This final judgment on the dress arrived at our apartment a few days later, when John brought home the photograph. In the picture my long, loose hair was wrong and frizzy in the humidity, and the nude hose I'd worn were dreadfully worse. I was not sexy, but shaggy; not "Red-Hot," but hangdog. Verdict? I had probably never looked beautiful in my designer dress: not in the store, not at home, not at the party. I lay down on the cold, granite window seat of our home office and cried because I was stupid, vain, heartbroken, and ashamed of all of it.

I tossed the picture in the trash.

FOR DAYS AFTER, I HID OUT IN THE APARTMENT, NURSING MY EGO and schlubbing around in tattered Lycra. The Red-Hot party was not the first of these fashion disasters. About four months before the party, John and I had met some of his colleagues for dinner, and I'd worn "something nice," only to meet everyone in pre-clubbing wear. More recently, there had been a staff barbecue. John billed it as a cocktail party, and in my black slacks and white blouse I'd matched the caterers (duh), not that it mattered, because thankfully all eyes were on Hattie, radiant in a onesie with spit-up on her sleeve. I'd felt like a cipher after that party, too: the arms that held the baby, the smile that framed the man.

Eventually, I snacked through all the dried fruit in the back of the cabinets and was forced to go out for groceries. I could have run down to our local Park-n-Shop for freakishly huge Mainland carrots and frozen dumplings, but for Hattie's sake, I opted for the largest, newest, best-stocked natural-foods grocery in the city.

It peeved me immensely that this store was located in the Landmark, Hong Kong's most extravagant retail arcade. It was perched atop von Furstenberg, Armani, and Michael Kors, as if healthy food and high fashion were not completely dissociative, as if indulging in thousand-dollar Jimmy Choos had something in common with paying twenty dollars for a jar of imported organic almond butter (which I had done once, by accident, and vowed never to do again). But there was no help for Hong Kong's insensitivity to the politics of luxury, and so it had become a habit of mine—after picking up organic produce flown in from across the planet—to gaze in those couture windows and dream of being in league with the women who wore clothes like this, women who wore scarlet ball gowns while picking heather on the moors or who lay draped across benches in leather dresses, holding gold revolvers just so. The shops in the Landmark seemed to promise I could be one of them—that the right product or garment or accessory could deliver me to myself at my imagined apex: clothed in riches, infinitely desired, mysterious, glamorous, and beautiful beyond compare.

It was while dreaming of this perfected self that I caught sight of my reflection in a shopwindow. I wore the insistently casual American uniform of frayed, ancient jeans and beaten-down canvas sneakers. My shirt had two food stains. The long, blonde hair that had been silken and flowing in arid California was a thick mass under John's blue LA Dodgers cap, and although I had applied concealer, mascara, and lip gloss in hopes of looking pulled together, fatigue and dissatisfaction showed at every seam.

You look like crap.

The inner Voice was a note higher and more strident than usual, but I had to agree with her about the crappiness. Reflexively, I found the small, soft lip of flesh encased in cotton knit hanging over the waistband of my jeans and pinched, not very gently.

Too bad you can't cut it off.

Usually, the Voice's sarcasm was funny. Today, it felt like a knife.

I set down the groceries and stood before that designer window, studying the person reflected there: five foot three, 120 pounds, thirty-two years old. Above my own reflection, I could see Hattie asleep in a backpack with her head lolling to one side, the picture of trust and good faith. Here I was, the mother of a child I once feared I couldn't have. Here I was in good health, on the adventure of a lifetime, and married to a loving husband who made enough cash that I could blow a few hundred dollars on a dress with an elastic waist. And still I spoke to myself like this? Still I yearned for something more? I wasn't satisfied?

No, said the Voice. *You aren't.*

Whose voice was it exactly, twisting the knife with such finesse? Whoever it was didn't like me and didn't like my clothes. Wanted me to want what I couldn't have. Never tired of pointing out my flaws, capitalizing on my fears, and pointing out the grievous distance between the inadequate putty of my face and body and the ethereal shimmer of true beauty. This Voice didn't ever want me to be happy, either, only to know how unhappy I really was. I longed to show my daughter a beautiful and compassionate world, but the inner Voice always put me up to demonstrating ugliness—dissatisfaction, ungratefulness, self-loathing, jealousy, unspoken anger, and fear.

That's just how women are, hissed the Voice.

I picked up my shopping bags again and left the Landmark, shaken.

Survey Question

Have you ever been bothered by how much or how often you criticize your appearance?

Sometimes	60%
Often	28%
Never	8%
Other	2%*

Hattie and I exited into the comforting roar of Des Voeux Road and plodded toward the entrance of Hong Kong's central public escalator. The world's longest, this escalator rises eleven city blocks and connects Hong Kong's hectic downtown with the Mid-Levels, a residential district that lies directly inland and sharply uphill. From its raised corridor I could peer into the windows of exclusive no-name kitchens

* These descriptive statistics represent the responses of women who took my Beauty Experiment Survey anonymously online. For more on my survey, see "About the Survey."

where underworld bigwigs were rumored to dine and down into wetmarkets where fish hearts were laid out for display—still beating—in Styrofoam trays. There were art galleries and antique dealers, reflexology parlors, slick and trendy bars, open-air teahouses, and soy-sauce breweries that seemed as if they'd been in business since the days of Albert and Victoria. Along both sides of the escalator were also hundreds of billboard advertisements, many for cosmetics, jeweled watches, designer clothing, spa services, and beauty salons. Commerce was a big game in Hong Kong, and women's luxury commerce often seemed to be the biggest game of all.

I let my eyes skip over the ads, feeling them push me toward the usual attitudes of improvement and correction. This manipulation had never bothered me before, but today it felt aggressive, violent even. It made me want to crumple and hide, but also hit back.

"I don't have to play," I thought. A years-long frustration took a sudden, surprising, shape. I could stop. I try and try, and it never works; I never become beautiful. So why not give up? What would happen if I simply stopped buying all those new clothes, new shoes, accessories, and hair products I think I need? What if I stopped using concealer, enhancer, and wrinkle corrector, and what if I even stopped hoping that they would work? How would I feel then? How would I look? Would doing that silence the nasty inner Voice? Would I start to feel a beauty apart from all the unattainable perfect femaleness around me . . . or not?

Coiffed and suited women clacked down the adjacent staircase on high heels, hurrying toward offices and lunch dates. It would be a big risk to dispense with a game everyone played. But the money, and the time, it could save—my God! I wondered what I might do with the extra minutes, and with all that money piddled away in a tube of lotion here, a pair of uncomfortable shoes there. Maybe I could become a good example for Hattie, instead of a bad one. But how long could I hold out? A week? A month? Could I do it for a year? The rest of my life? As I passed an advertisement filled with happy people in denim sportswear, my idea was brought up short. I had only one pair of jeans, the already worn-out pair I was wearing now.

You'd have to get some new ones before you started. Nice dark ones, without frayed seams.

There she was again, the Voice. My jeans were old, but they could hold out a few more months.

And there was a lot a person could do with sixty or seventy bucks besides spend it on a pair of jeans.* I knew that from traveling to Latin America and Africa; I knew that from living near Mainland China. Hong Kong itself has a legendary wealth differential between rich and poor.† It wasn't so apparent from the escalator, or as Hattie and I walked home along Bonham Road. Our own apartment building was a modern high-rise with an electric gate manned by a security guard and smiling doormen. The rear entrance, however, opened onto the much smaller buildings of Sheung Wan, a neighborhood that was once known, unbelievably, as the Chinatown of Hong Kong. It was filled with the kind of living quarters that rental agents never showed to expatriates—dark interiors, squatter toilets, and outdoor sinks. On nearby

* One supplement aimed at preventing an iodine deficiency in infants costs a mere fifty cents per dose every two years—a fraction of what most of us might spend on a tube of lipstick in an American drugstore.

† There are 1.26 million Hong Kong residents living below the poverty line, including one in three elderly residents. Many of these poor live in "cage homes," essentially a few lockable square feet of space in metal cages sheltered inside a large warehouse.

Eastern Street there was a methadone clinic that kept odd hours; no matter when Hattie and I walked to the park, there were always a few unhappy souls sitting on the curb with the stray cats, waiting.

The most disturbing example of Hong Kong's hidden poverty lived in the space between our building and a crumbling, two-story auto-repair shop next door. A mossy chasm of concrete and smashed bricks seemed a terrible place for a shuffling, arthritic elderly person to live, but all evidence suggested that a woman in a blue-flowered shirt slept in a person-size assemblage of cardboard boxes and tire retreads there, held together by clothespins and plastic bags. Through Hattie's Cantonese-speaking babysitter, Mari, I had asked this woman about her circumstances and gotten the story that she stayed with a daughter somewhere down in the housing blocks. Neither Mari nor I believed it: the shirt never changed. I didn't know what to do with this information now that I had it, so I just urged Hattie to smile and wave at Blue-Flower Shirt a lot, and we took her all our overflow baked goods.

The poverty of this gift of leftovers, the expense of my own groceries, the "necessity" of new seventy-dollar jeans, the odd evasiveness of my mental health and contentment—these things had never before seemed interrelated to me as I passed through our building's shiny, mirrored entrance many times a day. Today, they seemed inextricably enmeshed.

"*Mgoi,*" I said softly to the doormen, embarrassed by my own thanks as they held the way open for me.

When we got back up to our apartment on 19, I put the groceries away, dished out some O's for Hattie to eat, and turned on my computer, searching for data on what seventy dollars could buy.

ꝏ

AS A COLLEGE STUDENT, I'D SPENT A SEMESTER IN THE WEST African nation of Cameroon. One day, walking in Marché Melen—a neighborhood with minimal running water and open sewers—I'd witnessed something I never forgot, even as the raw discomfort of that semester faded over the years. A shoeless young girl had been standing in the dust at the side of the road, staring down at a slum vendor's selection of second-hand fashion and gossip magazines. It did not surprise me to see the sisterhood of physical beauty transcending culture—of course it did. What upset me was that *Glamour, Paris Match,* and *OK* were the girl's primary connection to Western women, this barefoot, slum-dwelling school-age girl living in a country plagued by AIDS, dysentery, government corruption, nonexistent health care, and rampant witch doctoring. It seemed to me, from my own schoolgirl's perspective, as if we were saying, "Got no sanitary supplies or plumbing to use them in? Got no sex education or condoms, and too few textbooks and shoes? Here, sweetheart, have a gossip magazine."

And now here I was twelve years later in my gated apartment—with almond butter in my fridge and an extravagant designer dress in my closet that just hadn't "worked" for me—and I couldn't find any stats on Cameroonian education. I did discover that the cost of a year's school fees in Zimbabwe was $1.5 million Zimbabwean. Roughly $200 American. Not too far from the price of a pair of designer jeans, two if they were on sale. The article I did find said that female high school students in Africa were resorting to prostitution to fund their educations. Schoolgirls in Hong Kong did that, too, but to fund their shopping habits.

I looked at Hattie; Hattie looked at me.

I had been . . . *dismayed* when I found out Hattie's sex before she was born. I felt instantly, even as I sat up on the examining table, that I was not equipped to be the mother of a girl. Nearly a year in, I still felt this way. Hattie would soon be a toddler, then a schoolgirl, then a young woman out in a confusing world, facing the same public messages and inner voice that were making me crazy. Would she, in time, become unconvinced of her own unique beauty? Would she hate her husband's pretty female colleagues? Would she buy dresses to make herself feel valuable and then turn despondent when they failed? When confronted by human tragedies like Blue-Flower Shirt and schoolgirl prostitutes, would she resort to the goodwill gifts of the economically powerless housewife: baked goods and smiles?

I watched my baby girl slide Cheerios across her tray. The intensity of her nine-month-old's absorption still amazed me. It also terrified me: whatever—and whoever—I chose to put in front of her, she would study intently, remember, and know.

Survey Question

How would you rate yourself as a "beauty role model" for a young girl?

Excellent	15%
Pretty good	46%
In the middle	24%
Pretty bad	8%
Terrible	2%
Other	2%

The Beauty Experiment

> Plainness has its peculiar temptations quite as much as beauty.
>
> —George Eliot, pseudonym of Mary Anne Evans, nineteenth-century British novelist

Hong Kong, March 2007

The idea for my beauty experiment was to gather up all my appearance accoutrements and chuck them, because they'd failed me. Out would go the makeup, the clothes, the pampered long hair, and the jewelry, along with the efforts of trying so hard to look right. Since I could never hit beauty's mark, why even aim? Why bother? I knew my definition of beauty was extremely limited; I didn't mean mountains, generosity, great choral works, or brilliant equations. But this was part of my problem—I fixated on looks, probably to the detriment of all the other beauty out there. If I pulled this weed that always tripped me up, in its place surely something else would grow. I'd paid lip service to the notion of inner beauty all my life, but certainly hadn't ever worked as pointedly or energetically on cultivating it as I'd worked on, say, my hair.

But could I really give all that crap up? For at least a year, if not forever?

No way in hell, sister, said the inner Voice.

Absurd. It was an early afternoon two weeks after the Red-Hot party, and Hattie and I were meeting Anne and her daughter Eva, at the park. I decided that when I explained my abstention-from-beauty idea to Anne, I'd characterize it as a joke. It cheered me to think of Anne laughing, and rightly so, at the idea of giving up concealer, mascara, new shoes, and clothes. "And what next?" she might ask. "Toilet tissue?"

Hattie and I rode down one elevator and then another to the back entrance. Blue-Flower Shirt was nowhere in sight. I pushed the stroller over concrete blocks, wheeled around the dog-piss hydrant, and crossed Eastern Street into King George Park, with its shady gazebos, concrete soccer pitch, and playground. When we caught up to Anne and Eva, the little girls flapped at each other from their strollers, and we women began to exchange that mundane, essential litany of details about snack volume and nap-time length. After a moment, though, Anne cried, "Wait!" and brought Eva's stroller to a halt.

"How was the big party?" she asked. "Did he like the scarlet dress?"

I'd told her all about my purchase right afterward, and had emphasized the long sleeves and luxurious feel of the velvet. Now, I looked across the soccer pitch at the cascading banyans opposite us, not meeting Anne's eyes.

"He said he didn't expect it to look the way it did," I said carefully. "I think he was expecting something plunging or something." I looked down, manufacturing some pressing business with my stroller's brakes. Was it possible that the dress could summon tears three times?

"Gordon Bennett!"* Anne exclaimed, as observant as she was tactful. "What does the man want? An eighteen-year-old tart or a wife?"

I sniffed.

"I just don't think they have any idea how hard it is to find something suitable in Asia," she went on. "Everything is cut for A-cup girls who don't weigh more than eight stone."

"I'm glad you'll never have to see what I saw in the dressing rooms," I said. "Hattie's lucky she slept through it." Remembering that baby-doll dress I'd tried in the local shop, I was able to laugh. We resumed our walk, exasperation and empathy pinging between us as the little girls toddled toward the playground.

By the time we headed back to the building, I still hadn't mentioned my foolish no-beauty idea. I was deeply grateful for Anne's feather-smoothing over the problem of the dress. But this also helped me realize how big that problem was. At the moment of confessing it, I'd switched to concealing. Something was really wrong with me here, something I was embarrassed to share even with a good friend. If I could muster some remove about myself and my situation, this was interesting.

After Hattie was in bed that night, I drank a little wine and wrote a few pages. I wrote about the dress, the frustration, and what it might be like to experiment on myself, giving up on one kind of beauty to find something else. When John got

---

* Gordon Bennett was a wealthy socialite-turned-journalist of legendary exploits and bad behavior. In 1930s Britain, his name became a more polite stand-in for the oath "*God blind me.*"

home around nine o'clock, I printed out my pages and handed them over.

This was a risky thing to do. When we'd become a couple, right after college, the juxtaposition of our backgrounds had been romantic. He was a dashing financial whiz with an artistic bent, and I was the nerdy liberal artist from Vermont. Together we rode camels in Mongolia, wrote a performance piece that was half short story and half sonata, and agreed to carrots-and-celery cleansing after every fried-oyster po'boy and Taiwanese oil-stick sandwich we shoveled down. Over time, however, we discovered serious vocabulary problems, especially when it came to our professions. John could not explain anything he was working on without defining multiple 101-level financial terms for me. ("What do you mean, 'What is principal?'" he might ask, purple with disbelief.) And while he could appreciate my stories about selling nasal tissue for cash, he had no grasp of the terms *process* or *constructive criticism* when it came to my writing. If he could put a piece down after the first three sentences, he did.

Neediness overwhelmed my ordinary reluctance that night, and as John sat at the table reading the pages, I hovered in the doorway, circling his approval—or dismissal—like a cat with a skittish mouse.

"You do think about this stuff a lot," he observed, not looking up.

"Too much," I said.

He read the printout without stopping, giving my pages the kind of attention he usually lavished on the *Handbook of Fixed Income Securities.*

"Are you really going to do it for a whole year?" he asked, looking up.

"I think it has to be that long, or it's just a waiting game. A test of my willpower. It's not making me live inside the decision."*

He nodded in agreement. "So you'd give up all this stuff for a year," he said, "and take notes. And then what? Write something about it?"

"I don't know what I'll do with it," I replied, not having gotten that far. The point of doing all this was me: my attitude and my ability to be a good role model. Right now, I was just happy he was interested.

"So how are you going to handle the gray areas?" John asked, twirling his pen and looking up, the light of analysis now burning in his eyes. "What about shampoo with conditioner mixed in?"

"Exactly!" I said. "What about tinted Chapstick?"

We considered.

"Tinted Chapstick would be sticking to the letter of the law," John advised, "but not the spirit."

"I think you're right. Maybe I should get a pen," I said.

Mixing my reformer's zeal with John's thirst for precision, we hammered out a set of rules for my experiment that night. We reasoned that because most men we knew didn't suffer from beauty craziness, it might be best for me to adopt a masculine approach to personal hygiene: just the basics. We also agreed that since I would not slather on three-quarters of a cup of wet-look gel in the morning (as did John), I would get to use sunscreen and facial moisturizer with sunscreen in it. We lived near the equator, and I wasn't prepared to risk skin cancer for this experiment. John agreed this was fair.

---

* Remarkably, I had never heard of any of the yearlong-stunt nonfiction projects when I conceived of my experiment in 2007.

The Rules

DURATION OF THE EXPERIMENT:

one year

DAYS OFF:

none

WHAT I COULD USE:

hand cream
deodorant
bottle of shampoo
bar of soap
sunblock and moisturizer
dental floss
toothbrush
toothpaste
wooden comb
scrub mitt
nail clippers

WHAT I WOULD TOSS:

undereye concealers: 3
pressed powder
blush
lipsticks: 5
lip glosses: 2
lip liner
mascaras: 3
eyeliner
eye-shadow compacts: 2
makeup remover
nail polishes: 11
nail-polish remover
collagen hand scrub
collagen facial masks
antiwrinkle apricot night cream
antiwrinkle retinol night cream
antiaging firming cream
anti-stretch mark massage cream
antibrassiness hair glosser
antifrizz hair serum
cleansing mousse
straightening hair gel
sparkly body powder
microdermabrasion kit
body butter
sunless tanner
hair-removal strips
depilatory lotion
razors
shaving cream
gel hair-removal kit and lotion
broken vanity mirror
schizophrenic scale

What I Wouldn't Use, but Could Keep for Later (Postexperiment):

earrings: 38 pairs
rings: 7
bracelets: 13
necklaces: 20
scented body powder (gift)
fancy skin-care set (gift)
hair lightener from overseas
manicure and pedicure kit
hair elastics and brushes
blow-dryer
butane hair straightener
perfumes: 3

As far as clothes, I would wear what I already had—no more shopping trips. Easy. I could also wear my wedding rings and a watch, but I lobbied for my tiny gold earrings, too, arguing that they'd keep the holes in my ears from closing. Whether those holes would really close was suspect, but I could feel panic fizzing under my breastbone as I realized just how many of my womanly potions and lotions would be thrown away.

"So what about Anne and Corinne and everyone?" John asked, leaning back in his chair at the dining table, as bemused as a college kid helping a friend vet a prank. "Are you going to tell them what you're doing?"

We went back and forth a while on this, John listening while I circumnavigated the living room, talking out the angles of disclosure. This aspect made me nervous, as it should have. Letting my friends in on the beauty fast would open the conversation and yield a lot of opinions. On the other hand, part of the experiment was to observe other women, and people who know they're being observed say and do what they normally wouldn't. I also didn't want to risk alienating the few friends I had. Was it bad policy to fight a battle publicly—and suggest that your own problem was one everyone shared? Was it any better to work on it privately, in secret? We agreed this was tricky territory and that I might have to try it out for a while secretly and see how it felt.

"And you, too," I warned John. "Think carefully about what matters to *you*, because you're gonna have to look at the eye bags, the acne, and the shaved head all year."

"You're going to shave your head?" John said, blanching, his tipped chair coming down.

I reveled in this quadrupling of spousal interest in my hair.

"I might."

"I guess if you think you have to," he said casually, returning to his accounting literature.

This was why I loved him. Why he drove me crazy. If I needed to shave my head, he'd be the last one to stop me—he'd had a college girlfriend do it once, no skin off his back, or so he'd let you believe. Sometimes I felt as if I were married to an elephant, an exquisitely intelligent creature with a brain and senses that were similar to mine, but not the same, and who might either be ignoring or misunderstanding or outwitting me, depending on the day and his mood.

"I think a shaved head would be counterproductive," I finally said. "It would draw attention to my looks when I'm really trying to get *around* looks."

"That sounds right," John agreed, noncommittally, but I thought he looked relieved.

The apartment was quiet a few moments. I thought the conversation was over, but then John ventured, very tentatively, "How about shaved legs? Shaved legs are nice."

"They are nice," I agreed. Noncommittally.

Snapshot: *Blind Spot*

New Jersey Suburbs, April 2011

It is early spring, and I live in New Jersey now. I have two children, not one, and the view out my window is a neighbor's clapboard house, not the busy waterway between Kowloon and Hong Kong. Even so, this morning, I can still see that woman-I-was in that nineteenth-floor apartment very clearly. I can see John with perfect clarity, changed out of his suit into an undershirt and sweats, an almost-emptied package of McVitie's digestive biscuits in his hand. I can see the green marble legs of the dining table and can almost feel how the wine dulled my frustration with myself but sharpened my desire for approval from my husband, from my daughter, and from the world.

As I type these memories—closing my eyes to hear our words and the tone behind them—I find a hole. There was another very important aspect to my experiment. The money. The savings jar. The donations. The do-gooding. The second part of my big idea was to keep track of all the money I would have spent on all things beauty related in a year, and then turn it over to some charity organization instead, something related to Blue-Flower Shirt or those schoolgirls in Zimbabwe and Cameroon. If anyone was qualified to help me flesh out, organize, and record the dollars and cents of these redirected beauty spending habits, it was John. Yet as I recollect this evening scene, I find I don't remember explaining the philanthropy aspect of my experiment to him. I didn't mention the way I planned to record every instance of consumerist desire in a little notebook, then eventually swap these desires for actual cash. I don't remember telling him about my still-vague plans for the money or showing him my save-as-I-go jar, a clear-plastic flip-top container emptied of its granola bars. When I turn this moment around and around in my mind, all I get is fog.

The things we forget can suggest what is unimportant, but also where our blind spots are, those moments when we don't even realize that we're ignoring, editing, or looking away from the ball. I think I've forgotten what was said about my philanthropy plan because that woman-I-was didn't want to talk to her husband about money. Despite both being . . . *thrifty* is the kind word for it, there were still a hundred ways in which our spending habits differed, a hundred values, preferences, and intentions that were not precisely the same. Why would the woman-I-was go near this known marital sinkhole and sour a husbandly approval so newly won?

She wouldn't. She would underplay the philanthropy, or keep it to herself. As the woman-I-am-now gazes into my teacup on this cold spring morning, I recognize the start of a troubling silence that went on to deepen and grow.

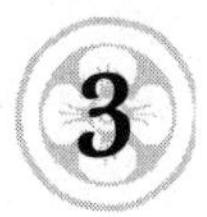

The Hair Questions

> Hair style is the final tip-off whether or not a woman really knows herself.
>
> —Hubert de Givenchy, French fashion designer

> If truth is beauty, how come no one has their hair done in a library?
>
> —Lily Tomlin, actress, comedian, producer

Hong Kong, March 2007

You can't cut it off, said the Voice. *And you won't.*

I stood sideways before the bathroom mirror that next morning, a Saturday, holding out behind me a fourteen-inch hank of reddish blonde hair. I swung it back and forth, then let it cascade reassuringly onto my shoulders. Throughout an awkward childhood, my hair had been my singular claim to poster-girl beauty. When my glasses were owlish and my limbs thick and blunt, I had good hair. It was silky, sunny-strawberry, and long even when I dressed myself in unflattering cutoffs and had a combative attitude. It was everything—sometimes the only thing—that I felt made me a sexually attractive female. I had suffered a bad bowl cut at age seven and went chin length for my middle twenties, but the short lengths were always the Beta—a test drive of sleekness but not my real hair identity. My real hair belonged in a Garnier Fructis commercial.

I faced front and pulled the hair into a tight ponytail, as if it were gone. The Voice spoke up.

Your nose is too big for that, and your chin is too weak. You don't look pretty.

Pretty shmitty, I countered, surprised at how good it felt to contradict the Voice. Maybe I was no longer trying to minimize my nose or maximize my chin; I was trying to give Barbie the finger. Plenty of women had done it by shaving or chopping their hair: Joan Jett, Sinead O'Connor, Sigourney Weaver in *Aliens,* Demi Moore in *GI Jane*—tough girls all! On the other hand, though, Brittany Spears had taken the clippers to herself in Sherman Oaks a month earlier, and images of her stressed and unhappy female baldness were still all over the place. In many cases, the identity a woman lost along with her hair was replaced by a more troubling public signal of disease, oppression, or rebellion. I thought of my college friend Elise, who'd shaved her head before leaving her difficult marriage and flying to Kauai to live on fifty dollars and the benevolence of the universe. It was not a good time in her life.

It wasn't toughness or trauma I wanted, but simplicity. Since arriving in Hong Kong, I'd been fascinated by the hairless Buddhist nuns I often spotted around and wondered if, when their brains were closer to the morning sun, they had clearer thoughts about the produce and tofu they were poking at roadside stalls. I could use some clear thoughts, some cranial warming.

I let the hair fall loose again and looked at the floor of the bathroom. The garbage can was close at hand, and my tools of depilation were ready for purging—the Veet home-wax strips (legs), the tweezers (chin), the razor (pits), and the Nair cucumber lotion (bikini line).

"Once you start," my mother had warned me of depilation, "you cannot stop." I was eleven the day she told me this and had just described to her the mortification of being the only girl in my circle of sixth-grade compatriots who did not shave her legs. Our ringleader was Shawna White, who had a sister in high school, and describing Shawna's daily tut-tutting finally broke Mom's resolve. She reluctantly handed over her electric shaver. The morning after my debut shave, I rode my bicycle to school bare-legged in a full skirt. Halfway there I began to wonder if I'd done something wrong with the shaver. I stopped my bike, rubbed my numb, smooth skin, and realized I could no longer feel the wind on my legs. If Ma was right, I never would again.

Now I saw this was bunk. I could reclaim my childish sensory pleasures and defy Shawna White if I pleased. But did I? It was hard to figure out whether *I* felt that it was antiempowered to shave or wax what nature gave me, or whether someone *else* felt that way, someone I read about once, or saw sunbathing on a European beach and decided was cool. What I did know is that whether I shaved daily or waxed monthly or dissolved my body hair into a stinky "cucumber and aloe" chemical mass just moments before plunging it into a chlorinated pool, it never felt very good.

You don't know hurt until John reaches out for your leg in bed and says, "Gross."

Fine. Body hair had a few pluses—skin sensations and the trapping of odorless, aphrodisiac pheromones—but it was also true that men generally had more body hair than women.* The kicker was that men generally had more hair than women of their same genetic makeup. As a Caucasian female married to an Asian male, the game was rigged against me. John had about sixteen hairs on one leg and seven on the other, nothing compared to the calf-Afro I'd produce if I abandoned all hair management. In addition, Hong Kong's daily temps provided shorts weather for most of the year, and the city seemed to have skipped over any notions of hippie culture or "barefoot beauty" and gone straight to eighties shoulder pads and neon geometry. An overly aggressive body-hair statement would not read as "liberated woman" or even "Scandinavian Euro-goddess" but as "insane and doesn't shower." I wanted to be revolutionary and free, but I did not want to go a year without sex or casual conversation.

Because I'd seen a few older Asian women with tiny amounts of underarm hair, I decided to work their groove and let mine grow. I dumped my razors and felt gleeful at the prospect of a year without stubble or the rashes it gave me. My upper legs and bikini line were *usually* covered, so I'd grow those, too. I figured I could handle a little lower-leg hair, but the full Caucasian calf-Afro was asking too much of Hong Kong, and me, so I put the home-wax strips back in the cabinet, to use for hair "reduction" every other month or so.

* There's an interesting theory about this, too: gender differences in body hair—particularly on the arms and legs—possibly stem from gender roles that helped early human societies thrive. Active male hunters needed more sweat glands and body hair to cool them down, whereas nimble-fingered female gatherers needed fewer.

I also had one further embarrassing—even shameful—choice to make. No woman likes to admit what crops up on chins, upper lips, out of beauty marks, or between brows, but hey, there they were on me, plucked all the same.

Absolutely not. No face hair. Nonnegotiable.

Oh, but come on! This was the really radical stuff; this was the bleeding edge! When I was in college, one of my professors invited the performance artist Jennifer Miller to visit. Her bit included showstoppers like juggling knives, but what totally upstaged the flashing steel was her *full beard.* Pretty/ugly/pretty/ugly/—the experience of looking at a bearded lady had been awesomely transgressive.* Although I lacked the hormones to pull off a full Paul Bunyan, I had a few follicles that might be counted on to shock and awe.

No.

Slowly, I put my tweezers back into the cabinet. I was no Jennifer Miller, yet. Possibly never would be. I felt substantially disappointed in my conventionality. Also, wicked relieved.

How I Handled the Body-Hair Question

lower leg:	at-home wax every two to three months
face:	pluck strays
armpits:	let grow
bikini area:	let grow
upper leg:	let grow
entire pubic area:	let grow
arms:	let grow

* Any search engine will yield two or three gender-bending images of Miller, or check out her current project: www.circusamok.org.

As for the head hair, the choice was clear, if not easy. I left the bathroom and pulled the camera out of its drawer.

"Get it from the back," I told John, going into the bedroom where the morning light would show the color better. "You don't need the rest of me, just get the hair."

He photographed my long hair, undamaged by chemicals, or even hairdryers, falling to my midback.

"Okay," I said. "Squiffy, here I come."

Squiffy was a unisex hair salon down the street where John got his haircuts for about seven US dollars. He felt it was an excellent deal because a brief shoulder massage was included in the price. The first day I went, I assumed the place had just been cleaned; later I learned it always reeked of lemony disinfectant. There was a glass tank opaque with algae, but it was inhabited; one giant orange fish eye peered through a gap toward a tilting check-in counter and its bowl of fused sesame candies.

"*Mgoi,*" I said to the woman at the counter, thanking and apologizing and requesting all at the same time. I was waved in to wait among the nearly twenty people already hanging around—it was hard to tell who was an employee and who a customer, but one thing was sure, I was the only Westerner in there. Everyone seemed to be wearing a smock, and everyone seemed to have a hairdo that was half-finished—spiky in front, long in back; curly in back, red in front. An elderly woman sat under a menacing, antique permanent machine, her hair rolled up into tens of black springy coils and pulled tightly away from her scalp, medusa-like. She was calm during this torture, reading a magazine.

The long-haired owner of Squiffy himself had a "do" that was puffy, layered, and looked bitten off at the ends. I nervously waived the massage, so he ushered me into his chair and listened with consternation to unintelligible Mandarin as I tried to convince him I did not want a cut like his, or like any of the cuts in the style books, but a sleek, simple man-cut. He argued with me, especially about the length of the sides. I wanted short, but he clucked disapprovingly and counseled long, so I could tuck it behind my ears. In the end, I just concentrated on the sound of the scissors as they hacked away fourteen inches. My efforts at detached equilibrium were undermined by an enterprising shampooist who rushed over and scooped up my golden locks the second they hit the floor. She double-bagged them carefully, then spirited them away to an upstairs break room, the better to preserve them—for sale to a wig maker, I guessed, although there might not be a big market for my hair color in Hong Kong.*

"Okay. *Yes!*" I told Mr. Squiffy with a tight, squeaky voice when he was done. "*Hen how.* Very nice. That is exactly what I wanted."

The cut was cheap but, because I was a woman, still double the price of John's haircuts. I paid, walked out, and kept my eyes firmly on the other people passing me as I walked home. I looked at the stoplight at the intersection of Caine Road, not the windows of cars passing, and I looked at the smooth, polished floor in the elevator, not the mirrored walls.

Back home, I played it cool.

"I just asked for a man-cut," I said lightly, running my fingers through bristly tufts. "He didn't believe me, though. He gave me these weird sideburns. Look." I drew the hair behind my ears forward, so it made a strange crescent shape on my cheek.

---

* Had I known about it that day, I would have collected my own hair and sent it off to Locks of Love, an organization providing wigs to children undergoing chemotherapy: www.locksoflove.org.

John snickered.

"It is kind of sixties Bauhaus," he said, turning me to the side, inspecting. Back in the States, where only select barbers knew how to deal with his coarse, straight Asian hair, John had lived through an array of haircutting disasters: shelf head, exposed cowlicks, and weird thinning techniques that left him with a modified mullet. He could spare empathy for a hideous do, but had less for what was only a new look.

"It's not that bad," he pronounced, petting my head as he assessed. "I realize it's a big change, but he did a good job. Nothing is sticking up or sticking out. You look like a regular person."

I nodded mutely.

"I'll give you twenty-four hours to stop looking at it," he added, and left me in front of the living-room mirror, transfixed by the strange, shorn woman there.*

When Hattie woke up from her nap, I expected tears. I was prepared for some big reaction akin to the family story my mom liked to tell about my two-year-old freak-out when Dad shaved off his beard. Instead, I got nothing: only average fretting and clinging and ordinary interest in a snack. Hattie was attached not to my hair, it seemed, but to my mothering. To me. I understood that I should be encouraged by this.

I was not. Six hours in, I was back in front of the bathroom mirror again, addressing the truth of dark roots, a big nose, and a weak chin. I'd threatened the Voice with nonfeminine and nonbeautiful, and here it was. I did not cry. Instead, I rummaged around for a pair of nail scissors and then savagely cut off the sideburns, nicking my ear. It took a moment, but

* In a study commissioned by hair-care products retailer TRESemmé, women spent, over the course of their lives, an average of seven months and fifty thousand dollars on their hair.

just as Mr. Squiffy had warned, the now too-short hair winged out on the sides.

The next day was a Sunday, and we'd made a date with friends to hike Dragon's Back, one of the most famous and best-loved hikes in Hong Kong. I'd been looking forward to this outing with my friend Kit and her family, but sleeping on my new haircut produced terrible bending and poofing that had to be wetted and slicked flat. This first-thing-in-the-morning labor sapped my enthusiasm completely. I tried not to think about my missing hair and slapped a visor over it. But while preparing the sunscreen and snacks, I caught sight of myself in the living-room mirror. With a hat on, the haircut looked sporty and fresh. Unexpectedly, I liked it. With that single change, the whole tenor of the morning shifted, as if some huge logistical difficulty had been removed. As I more cheerfully filled the water bottles and scouted out the shoes, I wondered just how often negative opinions like this complicated my tasks. Bad-hair days and good-hair days: maybe less about the hair than the head underneath.

During the hike, the wind was in our favor. There was none of the usual smog drifting in from Guangzhou. Once we gained the crests of the Dragon's Back trail, we could see straight down on two sides: to the east we looked down into Shek O, Hong Kong's sandy, easternmost bay, and to the south we could see out toward the islands of Tai Po. The baby girls, up in their backpacks, were delighted with this vista in the bright sun. With John carrying Hattie and the ocean breeze on my exposed earlobes, I felt doubly lightweight and radically unencumbered. I talked a blue streak to our friends all the way up the ridge. We were at the top before my girlfriend Kit got a word in edgewise. She'd noticed the haircut right away but now asked, "So what inspired the big snip-off?"

I had not yet decided what to say about my experiment, or even if I was committed to it.

"It's just more convenient," I said. "I felt like I needed a change. I feel like I spend too much time on my looks sometimes." It was a bland answer, but true.

Kit nodded thoughtfully, touched her own lovely chestnut ponytail, and said, "It's quite brave of you, really."

"Oh, I don't know about that," I replied, laughing, but her comment surprised me, and I was more quiet for the descent, thinking. I had to agree with Kit that there was something daring in my act. It was not brave in the way of women who had to cross minefields for food or medicine, but sure, yes, a drastic shift in appearance could change the way people treated you, which could alter your behavior in turn. A good haircut was an act of grooming, but a completely new haircut was an identity maneuver. This fact was never lost on all those long-haired women on makeover shows who got their hair cut by style experts: the farm girls and beauty queens of *America's Next Top Model,* and the sixty-year-old Texan trying to look like her twenty-year-old bombshell daughter. Of course, they cried and freaked out when they were shorn. They were being robbed of a beloved and functional identity in front of a television audience, usually against their will. But when you did that same thing to yourself—if that identity already felt like a ball and chain—then being rid of it felt like freedom.

Our trail ended at a small scenic beach in the town of Shek O. We headed for the burger shack at one end and unloaded the babies from their packs. John and I stayed at our table to keep them from eating too much sand, while Kit and her husband went off to order us all some dinner. I'd shouldered Hattie in the backpack for the last stretch, and now that the weight was off, I felt as if I might float away. The sun was low.

I whipped off my visor. It felt incredibly good to pull my fingers through my hair until it stood up on end. John smiled at me, knowing how it felt.

I looked around at the other patrons in the café and wondered if they saw someone less traditional and more daring than the person I'd been. Was I more likable and interesting, or less, and to whom? Maybe I was a person who ate burgers with a knife and fork, or someone who told great jokes. I took off my shoes and socks and looked out toward the ocean—another shimmering expanse that seemed limitless and unknown.

Snapshot: *Winter Fur*

New Jersey Turnpike, May 2011

It's a Saturday, and John and I are taking the kids on a car trip. I'm the p.m. driver in our family, so this morning I sit in the passenger's seat and enjoy the pastel landscape: wet Pennsylvania farmland, hemmed by white ash trees in bloom. We have the windows cracked, and I can feel the warm spring air against my neck and ears, just as I did that long-ago day of the hike along Dragon's Back. I still keep my hair short, although it's no man-cut. With two kids constantly in tow, I hardly need—or have time for—a luxurious banner advertising my female sexuality. What I do need is a chance to doze and recharge every six weeks in a stylist's chair.

I'm not committed to this look forever, though. I recently spotted a beautiful woman in her fifties with luxurious gray hair to her waist and wondered if that might one day be me:

sexy in the years after fertility, attractive in an openly mature way, my grays a crown of wisdom, not a liability of age. As silly and self-congratulatory as it sounds, my experiment helped me learn to dismiss archaic rules of style ("hot chicks have long hair; older women have short") in favor of a hair identity sensitive to my own changing taste, environment, and sense of what's practical.

During the cold months of a New Jersey winter, I've also been able to do, on home turf, what I wasn't able to in Hong Kong. I have my feet up on the passenger's seat, and the hair on my ankles, peeking out now between my pant legs and socks, is completely grown in. I haven't shaved or waxed since October. Since they are so in evidence this morning, I ask John how he feels about the attractiveness of my winter-fur lower legs.

"On a scale of one to ten, how bad are they really?" I say. "Ten is the worst."

He gives it three seconds' consideration and then answers cheerfully, "Seven."

"Yeah," I say lightly. "That's what I figured." I look out at the red barns and telephone poles, not as bothered by this as I might once have been.

Through my research and the responses of my survey takers, I've come to see depilation as an age-old human quirk, one inextricably tangled up with more than one development in human culture.* But I also have reason to believe that with practice, a little female body hair can be tolerated

* In a 2003 *Guardian* essay, Mimi Spencer called depilation "the battle that feminism lost," suggesting that modern women have capitulated to a Victorian phobia of mature female body hair. But notables the world over, including Greek poet Ovid, have given hair-maintenance edicts for *both* sexes, generally for reasons of hygiene. Today, running water and soap do more for cleanliness than shaving, but the prevalence of tick-borne illnesses in the United States presents women and men a new reason to break out the razors, especially in the summer.

in public—by men and, perhaps more important, by women themselves.

Survey Question

Is a woman's sexual desirability jeopardized by having more body hair than her partner?

	Women	Men
Yes, quite a bit	37%	52%
Yes, a little	20%	18%
Not really	27%	15%
No, not at all	6%	5%
Other	8%	7%

Survey respondents' rank of body parts most important to depilate:

1. Lower legs and armpits
2. Face
3. Bikini area
4. Upper legs
5. Entire pubic area
6. Arms

Percentage of respondents who've depilated their entire pubic area at least once: **38%**

At a recent playgroup for Hattie's younger brother, Orson, we moms were standing in a friend's kitchen, sipping coffee and kvetching about projects we'd had to abandon and things we no longer cared so much about getting done. I pulled up my pant leg to show off my winter fur, and there were audible gasps all around.

"Ooooo, can I touch it?" one friend asked, and although she was being silly and we all were making light, she did reach out for a quick stroke. Even though every one of us would have agreed leg hair was an incredibly minor concern in the context of parenting, partnerships, economic turmoil, and careers unwound, my ungroomed legs were still showstoppers, were still knife-juggling bearded ladies. It's still a big question for most of us: if we go out imperfect, in public, will *we* stop the show?

My experiment answered that one neatly for me: yes, but only for the split second it takes everyone to realize it's no big deal. In a world where most of us have learned to smoothly tolerate visible thongs and butt cracks, tongue piercings, and all manner of appalling comb-overs in public, female leg hair is hardly offensive. Reverse the genders, and our fear of leg hair seems absurd: although not everyone loves to kiss a man with a beard, and most men do shave, a five o'clock shadow is perfectly acceptable in the grocery or at the playground, even sexy. As funny as it sounds, my experiment rid me of my own female hair shame. Depilation does sometimes end up on my to-do list, but if I have to make a playground run on an unseasonably hot spring day in shorts and my fully grown-out winter leg muffs, it might take a bit of backbone, but the world does not end. Hair matters, but it's not nearly as big a part of my identity as I believed or, perhaps, as big a part as arbiters of traditional femininity or liberated femaleness would have me believe.

A case in point: we're trying to sell our house, so John and I have cooked up this all-day car trip for the kids to keep them occupied while our real-estate agent hosts an open house. I have spent the past two weeks on the suburban home owner's equivalent of last-minute hair management: whacking weeds, trimming woolly shrubbery, touching up paint. After two years in New Jersey, we are moving again, this time to Boston, and facing the job of establishing identities again—as a family, as a couple, and as individuals: woman, man, little girl, and baby boy. When I prop my feet up on the dashboard, it certainly isn't my ankles—hairy or not—that reveal anything meaningful about me. The more revealing canvas is the one I now massage with my fingertips, releasing tension in my forehead and loosening worry around my mouth, as we speed ahead into another season of growth and change.

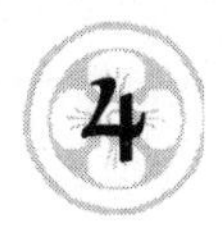

Two Half-Moons of Peach Paste

The most exhausting thing in life is being insincere.

—Anne Morrow Lindbergh, author, aviator, environmentalist

Hong Kong, April 2007

It wasn't all as easy as that first hike. I missed the glimmer of jewelry and the optimism of a new outfit more than I'd expected. Every day I fretted that my eyes lacked focus and my lips were wan and thin. I wasn't always happy with my haircut, either. With it, I sometimes felt ugly, but more often just plain: unbeautiful, unremarkable, and uninteresting to the eye. I sometimes felt, not masculinized, nor made less female, but less *feminine*, and by extension less traditionally sexy. The sporting-goods store I'd worked in before moving to Hong Kong had been staffed mostly by lesbians, and I'd developed an envious appreciation of those fellow saleswomen who wore simple polo shirts with turned-up collars and spiky haircuts. But without the sexual orientation, Italian shoes, or German eyeglasses to back up my own haircut, I did feel depleted of some important piece of attractiveness, something I needed to get along in the world.

For nearly a month, I dragged an oppressive sense of plain Janeness around with me, a sense that doubled when I left the house, something I did less and less. I found a reason to skip Hattie's regular Friday baby group and agreed to go for exercise walks with Anne and another neighbor, Grace, only because we'd already shared birthing war stories that were far uglier than a sallow face or bad hair.

But like Kit, Anne and Grace were curious about my haircut and recent change. Now that I'd really gotten started, I wanted to give them answers as to why, but the ones I had didn't make much sense even to me.

"I'm thinking of getting one of those headbands," I told them one morning as we shoved our strollers uphill. "The pink ones you put on newborns. Just so you can tell I'm female."

"It's not so bad as all that," Grace said kindly, biting her lip.

"No, actually, I just love Hugh Grant so much I'm trying to look like him. 'Hi, ladies,'" I said suavely over the stroller handles. "'Ignore the breasts, and you'll see I'm incredibly charming.'"

Anne cracked a smile.

"I've decided to call my look 'the Momnisexual,' too," I went on. "Like a sister to the metrosexual. It's a look that says, 'I'm not trying to be pretty, yo, look where that got me—strapped to this kid 24/7 and trying to stay sane.'"

I wasn't ready to take my act to Vegas, but owning—and outing—my own critique certainly lessened its sting.

Funny bone, n.: A handy bit of psychic anatomy that pretty girls rarely need but the rest of the human universe has developed in spades.

ABOUT A MONTH INTO MY EXPERIMENT, I CAUGHT A NASTY TROPICAL flu. It normally would have been dispatched by three days under the covers, hot liquids, and some whimpering, but this healing cocoon was not available to me. John was away, and Hattie needed my constant attention. Relatives and friends lived across eight thousand miles of ocean, and our part-time babysitter was available only on appointed days. Most notably, John and I had chosen not to do what many families in Hong Kong considered a necessity: hire a live-in Filipina or Indonesian maid.

It was a decision I struggled with daily. My reasons were mostly personal: my father had been raised by a Filipino houseman, while my grandmother entertained her bridge club and pressed a bell under her foot when she wanted the martinis refreshed. It was a world I'd been raised to despise, and the moment I was enveloped in the expatriate bubble, I'd caught the scent of gin and ironed sheets. But while having a live-in servant looked awkward from the point of view of family history and social justice, from an economic standpoint it was a no-brainer.* What an amah gets paid monthly is less

* The cost of an American day care can start at $1,200 per month, whereas the legal minimum wage for foreign domestic workers in Hong Kong is $498 per month, usually including a room. The legal minimum wage for other kinds of workers in HK is $716 per month. There are approximately three hundred thousand domestic helpers or amahs from the Philippines, Indonesia, Nepal, and other countries working in Hong Kong, and while many legal protections for them have been established, amahs are still denied applications for permanent-resident status after seven years of residency. Interestingly, the female employers of domestics are often among the champions of their rights.

than half the cost of a month's tuition at an American nine-to-five day care, and as an inexperienced work-from-home parent with a busy spouse and no family around to rely on, I could have used the help.

The most acute ramification of this decision was that I felt like I hadn't slept in a year. My periods of nighttime unconsciousness were more like blackouts—reality cut out for a moment and then came back three or four hours later, with me no more rested, no more cogent. I had tried a whole bookshelf full of sleep-training techniques, but Hattie would do what Hattie would do: she was both owl and lark. John did what he could: he offered me an occasional Saturday-morning sleep-in, but he didn't have the breasts to effectively sub in for nighttime feedings. The dirty secret of this sleep-deprivation triangle was that *I* also did what I would do: I would not turn off the light at eight or nine o'clock in self-defense, but insisted on reading, working, or thinking into the night, feigning ignorance of morning's reality: nausea, self-recrimination, and despair.

The physical reality of "sleep debt" is that hours of lost sleep must be repaid in full. For example, one good night's sleep of eight hours does not make up for several days or months of only getting four. Lost sleep hours are carried over and become bricks around one's neck as much as monetary debt. The higher this sleep debt mounts, the more it inhibits creativity and learning, thrashes the immune system, increases sensations of pain, makes one more prone to violence, drastically worsens the sedative effect of alcohol and other narcotics, and encourages indifference to danger. Seventy-two consecutive hours of lost sleep can make a person collapse; the approximate amount of sleep lost by the parent of a new baby in the first twelve months is 350 hours.

I'd never heard of sleep debt during my first year of motherhood and so didn't always connect my poor sleeping habits with their effects: chronic nausea, migraines, and forgetfulness. I often felt despair, rage, hysteria, and confusion. I couldn't enjoy things I usually loved, had a sense of hopelessness that magnified as the day went on, and experienced hair-trigger outbursts of frustration (door and cabinet slamming). One of the most sinister aspects of sleep debt is that a person becomes habituated to it, noticing it less as it increases to more dangerous levels. Despite my symptoms, I was mostly habituated, until I got sick.

During my three days of flu, my fatigue was like a panicky thirst. It was the only thing I thought about, sleep the only thing I wanted and something I was almost prepared to do anything to get—hire six amahs, leave John and go back to the States, take Hattie down to the doormen and leave her there indefinitely. I didn't do these things, nor could I bring myself to trouble Anne—she didn't have an amah either, and if she caught the flu from us, I would have doubled the misery. Instead, I lay on the couch, drifting in the purgatory of half-sleep, neither being a parent nor calling someone else to sub in. Hattie ate the toddler equivalent of dry cat food while sitting in front of DVDs set to repeat. Although my experiment did not cross my addled mind, I followed all my rules to a T: no makeup, no mirror time, and I accessorized my old bathrobe with a puke bucket.

Recovery posed a new challenge. When I rose from my stupor, showered, and dressed, it was a Friday. There was an afternoon meeting of Hattie's regular playgroup, a perfect opportunity to free the poor kid from my exclusive company and the stinky apartment. But the woman looking back at me in the mirror belonged in a morgue. Her violet undereye bags bloomed two inches wide. This would be my very first public group appearance au naturel, and this sickroom mess was the face we'd be taking along.

You know what to do, the Voice said.

I did know, but my trusty wand of concealer no longer stood at attention on the back right corner of my vanity. There was no bottle of creamy pink perfecting lotion, either. There was also no brightener, no tightener, no tinted sunscreen, nothing at all for correction or improvement except a bottle of hand lotion I'd gotten free from the maternity ward that smelled like toilet-bowl cleaner. Despite the fact that all my flesh-toned "foundations" sweated off in about an hour and gave my wrinkles a nice chalky definition, I usually slathered them under my eyes and over my blemishes daily, or at least whenever I went out. I didn't wear these half-moons of peach paste to look good or pretty, either, but just to help me pass as normal: healthy, alert, in this case simply alive. With makeup on, I felt as if no one could see that I ate peanuts and Goldfish for dinner, that Hattie's crying made me want to punch a wall, or that sleep was a boat that left nightly without me. Going without this cosmetic prosthetic to an offi-

Survey Question

How often do you wear makeup now?

Never	6%
Occasionally	36%
Regularly	34%
Every day	18%
Other	3%

cial meet-up would feel like going out in public topless, or at least without a bra.

The sensation of nakedness would be exaggerated by the location of the playdate, too. It wasn't being held at a kiddie gym, but would take place in the kids' area of a private club, a club with an excellent restaurant overlooking a members-only marina. I'd been a caterer-waiter in fancy homes and clubs for years and wasn't wholly intimidated by exclusive places like this; it was just that I usually felt like I should go in through the service entrance near the trash compactor and start rounding up stray glasses. Whatever. It would all be fine; we should go. I gathered our paraphernalia, and we went down to the street and caught a cab.

It was a long ride to the south side of the island, over a hill and back down into Aberdeen, a port village whose proportions always made me wince. The tiny shacks up in the hills were stripped of their views and dwarfed by the massive concrete apartment blocks all crowded down at the water's edge. The road was at the waterfront, too, with the parks tucked into sooty underpasses. I had an ongoing beef with the modern Chinese aesthetic that allowed utility, efficiency, and commerce to trump everything else, including human beings and natural landforms. But who was I to judge, really? Here *I* was today, headed to the Aberdeen Marina Club in a look that clearly fell on the wrong side of the ugly line, yet I expected (hoped) the world to find some value in me. I'd never thought about the ethical component of aesthetics, but as we zipped smoothly through Aberdeen's crowds on an elevated road I considered an eyesore, it occurred to me that beauty was sometimes just a way to suggest the concerns of one group were more important than the concerns of another, and "good taste" just one of the hundred human ways to exclude. It pricked my conscience to realize how often I let visual beauty trump other worthy considerations. Possibly, I could think more about this. Possibly, I should adjust.*

As we drew closer to the club, I held Hattie's hand and pointed things out through the taxi's windows: a stadium and a helicopter in the sky. Attending to her made me wonder if curious glances would move toward my belly or if I'd be offered places to sit down. Pregnancy was the only truly acceptable reason for a woman to look unkempt and overwhelmed in Hong Kong, and any failing could be happily attributed to it—fatness, thinness, fatigue, eczema, bad hair, weird clothes. I bit my lips and pinched my cheeks, urging color into them as we pulled up in front of the club. We got out and I paid the fare. Twelve US dollars for a half-hour ride—arguably a beautiful thing. I nodded at the club's uniformed doormen and urged Hattie up the plush stairs.

"Hi there, you!" said Corinne, the outing's hostess, dumping her diaper bag on the floor and giving me a big cheek kiss. She had been one of the first people I met in Hong Kong, and she handed out invitations the way she handed out boxes of raisins—to any lost soul who needed them. Like me. "Great to see you, missus!" she said.

"Phoebe and Hattie!" said Kit, our friend from the hike. "We've missed you girls!"

"Oh my God, look at the hair!" exclaimed another friend who had short hair of her own. "It's wonderful!" She turned my chin and frowned approvingly. "Really, I like it so much better. Very chic."

* Said Leo Tolstoy, "It is amazing how complete is the delusion that beauty is goodness."

I could barely believe it. No one asked if I'd been down to Hell and back that morning. No one pinched me to see if I was alive. No one so much as glanced at my midsection, suggesting that my friends were maybe a hundred times kinder, more wonderful, and less concerned with my eye bags than I'd dared imagine.

It was a new, encouraging variety of embarrassment I felt as I tucked our two pairs of shoes into a tidy yellow cubby and then trailed after as Hattie ran to play with her buddies. I'd been afraid of what, exactly? That my friends would stick out their tongues and turn their backs on me? That they would really say, and really mean, what my own interior Voice threatened they would:

Your apartment is too small, your dishes are too plain, you don't have a maid, you can't make tea properly, your hair looks like a portobello, and your face is a mess, so I can't be friends with you!

As I reengaged with the living world, my concern about flu face receded. Left in its place, however, was an unexpected flicker of disappointment. This was a second surprise. I realized that I'd half *wanted* to be right about the female tendency to judge, shun, cold-shoulder, or sneer. There was grist in that. But against acceptance and unconcern . . . what weapons were there?

"Their kids' stuff isn't too good," I overheard one of our group say. "I wasn't impressed with the selection."

We'd begun discussing the inevitable: the hoopla surrounding the opening of a new department store in Central.

"I think it was just picked through already," said another. "We went early Saturday, and there was a line out the door by the time we left. With security guards."

"They have really cute knickers on the second floor," said Kit. "Cheap thrills."

"For kids?" asked Corinne.

"No, for me!" said Kit. "Can't I wear cute knickers anymore?"

Everyone laughed, and I laughed along, heartily, hoping to make up for what I feared was an obvious silence. I'd seen the lines, too, and had peeked in the new store's windows. The things on the mannequins were perfect for a lifestyle of playground outings and greasy, clutching fingers, but I had not gone in and would not be able to for a year. I'd anticipated giving up cute underpants, but suddenly I was feeling a new panic.

In Hong Kong, shopping talk was something of a national sport, earning its own newspaper sections like traffic or the weather. For men, this shopping talk was a pleasurable hobby: they could openly suggest tailors, jewelers, and electronics stores to one another. For women, it was much, much more. Both the YWCA and the American Women's Association sponsored newcomer events featuring shopping outings as a great way to meet new friends. (I had gone on one myself the month before Hattie was born.) Once you lived inside our wildly diverse international expatriate culture—a wholly female one in which husbands or partners rarely appeared—talk of stores and goods and prices could be steadfastly relied on for establishing common ground ("Did you go yet?"), as backdrops against which to field social or moral inquiries ("Tell me if you can believe this. She turns to me at the checkout and says . . . "), and to evoke sympathy and comprehension ("I just find it so hard to find gluten-free anything here!"). Whether the subject was cute underpants, effective skin care, useful baby equipment, cheap airfare, or cool hotel packages, shopping talk jumped right over socioeconomic and national lines. It bridged difficult territories like divergent parenting philosophies or opposing political views and dependably brought women together. Many times, I'd been grateful for the way it railroaded other subjects I was less comfortable with, like live-in helpers, wakeful babies, feelings of isolation, and preoccupied spouses.

As the department-store conversation went on, I decided I could tell no one about my beauty experiment until it was over. No matter how well I might explain it, publicly refusing to shop or talk about shopping in a retail mecca like Hong Kong would seem unforgivably pretentious and self-righteous. It would make my friends feel bad, or at least self-conscious, about a lingua franca we all took for granted. I could handle a year without concealer, but a year of awkward silence I could not do to any of us.

Surprise number three: beauty "freedom" was not as simple as I'd imagined. I could make any decision or follow any abstract principle I wanted, but emotionally and socially, I was already bound in a web, a web that provided connections I didn't want to jeopardize. I had been sure that I would feel more honest without makeup. Instead, I felt that I had traded one concealment for another.

Snapshot: *Unconcealed*

Warwick Hotel, Philadelphia, 2011

Today I am standing at the mirror in a hotel room, getting ready for my cousin's wedding. I took a shower early in the morning to save time and am already dressed: a pair of wide-leg cream trousers that I've been wearing to spring parties for years and a silky blue tank. The outfit is nothing fancy, but it is pulled together, and it fits. I brush my teeth and stroke my hair back so I can really see my face. I have a stress zit brewing at the corner of my mouth, and staring at it, I have a brief, sharp craving for concealer. Weddings, like other big family events and school reunions, require positive and triumphant news, not the uncertainty, stress, and doubt I feel about this move we are making. Immediately after this wedding, I will hop on a train north, to Boston, where I'll be scouting out neighborhoods, looking at rentals, and trying to find a place for our young family to land. Still, I don't even scrounge in my overnight bag because I know it isn't there. No concealer.

The last time I bought some was for my brother's wedding, in October 2008. John, Hattie, and I were in the midst of the international move back to the United States; John stayed behind, completing work projects and packing up in Hong Kong, while Hattie and I went ahead to my parents' home in the Southwest. I was six months pregnant with our son, Orson, at the time and suffering from sciatica. I was also panicked about finding a pediatrician, heart specialist, ob-gyn, home, car, and preschool in New Jersey in very short order. Hattie was potty training, or, rather, regressing. My beauty experiment was long over, but as my brother's wedding day approached, I bought concealer for the first time in more than a year, telling myself, "I never claimed to give it up forever." I knew, though—swiping it on, patting it in, repeating the process to build up accretive layers—that something was up. *Everything* was up. I was terrified. I was lonely, anxious, and, above all else, exhausted.*

* In isolated, bored, or stressed animals, excessive grooming is a known anxiety reliever, sometimes culminating in self-harm. Possible links between this finding and human grooming and self-harm behaviors are staggering and only beginning to be explored.

Instead of tossing my fourteen-dollar concealer in the trash, I called John. I told him that every night I lay in bed awake imagining plane-crash scenarios, fearing that our family would never unite. I explained that Hattie's jet lag had already lasted a full week. And I confessed. "I screamed at her," I whispered to him. "I told her to shut up."

John knows something of sleep deprivation and sleep debt himself. He reminded me to take short naps and long walks, put lesser tasks aside, and be patient with all the human beings I was juggling: mom, kid, fetus. He said he would be there soon, and in a few days' time, he was. I still wore concealer to my brother's wedding but not without awareness—concealer was a crutch, a signal of symptoms. It might be easy to slather two half-moons of cheerful peach paste under my eyes, but this did not resolve my fear or correct a substantial sleep debt.

Since my experiment, I've thought a lot about why I wear and have worn makeup and why other women do. My survey led me to suspect that many women—while okay with makeup generally—are less enamored with the *degree* of correction and mask wearing they feel compelled to perform.* The vast majority of my respondents had a cosmetic they'd like to scrap. I've also learned more about what goes into most makeup

---

* *Today Show* anchors Kathy Gifford and Hoda Kotbe were challenged by Rosie O'Donnell in 2010 to go without makeup during their national broadcast. "I feel like it's the dumbest thing we've ever done," said Gifford, who had a classic anxiety dream beforehand. Kotbe admitted that she also "kept waking up in the middle of the night. I didn't think this was a big deal until I realized that I don't even go running without lipstick on—because you never know who you're going to see." The show's own makeup artist, Mary Kahler, said "[Makeup] helps hide the fact that these women don't get much sleep—they are so busy, not only doing the show, but doing so many things afterward. They are constantly on the go and they have to look fresh even though they're going full speed ahead every minute."

through various watchdog websites and recent books. America's cosmetics industry is less regulated than sister industries in Canada, the European Union, and Japan, and few of us really know what we're smearing on our faces. Particularly at risk of being affected by some of these hazardous ingredients are women of reproductive age and teen girls.

Survey Questions

Can you name more than one ingredient in your most essential cosmetic?

I can't even name one	43%
No	36%
Yes	20%

Which cosmetic would you be happiest to throw in the trash and never have to wear again?

Foundation	25%
Lipstick or liner	12%
Concealer	11%
Mascara	10%
Blush	8%
Eye shadow or liner	5%
Other	9%
None	17%

So why do women wear makeup despite these or other reservations? Many of the women I surveyed wear their favorite cosmetic for the same reasons I used to slather on the concealer: to make them look healthier or conceal a problem or to make them look less tired. But even more women wear their favorite cosmetic to look "prettier or more feminine," a finding that suggests the unaltered female face doesn't have these qualities—or doesn't have enough of them for our tastes.

It's a bit like preferring the album to the live show, or the margarine to the butter. In a post-postmodern world like ours, this cultural preference for the artificial would be less strange if it didn't apply to women's faces only, but it does. I think about this taste for the hyperfeminine and all it entails when I imagine Hattie's future. Will I have to carefully police the contents of her lotions and potions throughout her adolescence, since the Food and Drug Administration won't? Will public concern over sleep deprivation ever shift from the public embarrassment of napping air-traffic controllers to the private tragedy of millions afraid to admit we're exhausted, overtaxed, and otherwise unable to keep up? I hope so. Most of all I hope my daughter will love the face and female identity she has—and feel comfortable with the window it gives into the reality of her woman's life. I hope she will believe, as I do now, that my own plain, real female face is neither mute nor invisible nor somehow inadequate, but interesting and expressive in its own right.

Today, in this Philadelphia hotel-room mirror, I look exactly my age: thirty-six. I look exactly my status: person with no time to use pore cleansers. You can see my mortgage in my forehead and professional insecurity at the corners of my eyes. Around my mouth, you can tell I've eaten bitter crow, screamed obscenities, and lost friends. But I got seven and a half hours of sleep last night because I didn't paint my nails, didn't rejigger my outfit at the last minute, and didn't wax legs that no one will see. I understand that my ability to deal with the stress in my life depends not only on alertness—caffeine can give me that in spades—but also on a more buoyant undercurrent of calm and well-being that can't be faked.

"You ready, Phoebe?"

It is my parents, who call to me through the door, not John. We could have booked a sitter and both gone to this wedding, but for a family under strain, this is the better choice: John gets time to be number-one caregiver for his own kids; I get a break from domesticity and time to connect with extended family. Making mildly unconventional choices in one realm of my life has made it easier in others, too.

Because this *is* a wedding, that most traditional and conventional of family parties, I add earrings to my outfit and sweep on some natural mascara and lip gloss. These days, I do sometimes enhance my appearance, but almost never do I conceal. Along with its opacifying properties, my cosmetic foundation contained dangerous toxic agents: false optimism and unrealistic ideals. If the world didn't see my fatigue and strain, then they weren't really there.

The Day I Covered the Mirrors

No woman wants to see herself too clearly.

—MIGNON MCLAUGHLIN, JOURNALIST, AUTHOR, AND EDITOR OF *GLAMOUR* MAGAZINE

HONG KONG, APRIL, MAY, AND JUNE 2007

Back during our first days in Hong Kong, John and I chose the thirty-five-story Bon Point building to live in, possibly because it was so easy to see ourselves there. During our tour, I'd found my own reflection dazzling in the reflective glass doors with gold chrome handles and in the polished stone floors. I also met myself in the mirrored elevator lobby, the mirrored elevator, and inside the flat itself: the baths were amply mirrored, the bedroom had a waist-to-ceiling mirror barely overpowered by a faux-snakeskin headboard, and if it were cleared of furniture, the living-dining area might have passed for a small dance studio.

"They do help," I'd said to the real-estate agent during the tour, meaning the mirrors gave an elegant but small apartment a needed boost of space and light.

Only on the day we moved in did I recognize the downside of this reflective arrangement. When I left the apartment, there I was, hunched over and adjusting Hattie's collar. When I rode the elevator, I was there in the doors, talking to a neighbor. When I walked through the lobby, my reflection flickered along behind, and when I returned, the reflection tromped in, too, lugging groceries and smoothing humidity-puffed hair. Inside the apartment, I was everywhere—frowning and examining the rapid swelling of my own abdomen in pregnancy and then its maddeningly slow shrinking. I stared at the baby I held in my own arms and wondered, *Who is this person?* I meant Hattie, but my gaze inevitably swerved back to me: who was this dour woman with the brow wrinkle and the infant? And what was she doing in Hong Kong?

Because my reflection was around so much, we became a team. We watched ourselves change diapers (stomach roll pronounced with these pants, neckline too low on this shirt), and we checked ourselves out while on the phone (weak chin, left is the better side). We hassled ourselves for picking the underwear out of our cracks, and if our posture was poor, we straightened up. We pointed out our undesirable aloneness when John was off in Tokyo or Seoul. We were models of reliability for each other: if one was chipper, both were perky; if one was sunk, we both went down.

I'd grossly underestimated how much I'd invested in this bizarre mirror relationship until John and I left the apartment for a midwinter trip, just a few weeks before the Red-Hot party.

Surrounded by good friends and Balinese water palaces, I left my reflection in the bathroom, over the sink with a stinky drain. There was retribution, however, when we got back. My reflection didn't greet me with the face of relaxation and inner peace, but met me with obvious travel fatigue and wrinkles deepened by too much sun and laughter.

The relationship with my reflection had soured further since the beginning of my experiment. As if I'd done her a personal wrong, my teammate glowered at me daily. I tried to avoid her gaze by busying myself with Hattie or by hiding out in the kitchen for an hour or so—even the worst interior designer knows better than to mirror the kitchen. This dysfunctional relationship crescendoed one evening in late April, as I was getting ready in the mirror for a friend's bachelorette party, or hen's night.

This event was my second night out on the town since I'd begun the experiment nearly two months earlier. The first had happened when Corinne invited me to the theater. Ignoring my mirror companion entirely, I'd worn the day's playground outfit to the performance—pilled navy sweater, brown cords, sneakers. My inner Voice had protested, screeching, "*You got that sweater at Goodwill!*" but I was early and did fine in the lobby, even when Corinne turned up looking fabulous in a dark silk blouse, low heels, and the kind of silver jewelry that suggests you are queen of a small island. Then she handed me a pass, and we went into a VIP area with people in cocktail attire. Whether these people actually started deriding me or not, my inner Voice had no trouble passing along their disdain: *That one is saying, "Egad, Americans,"* she whispered, *and that one over there thinks you look like you just came from changing a diaper*. Actually, I had. At the intermission, the Voice had this to add: *You should have worn black. At least no one would have noticed you.*

Black always felt funereal to me, especially at parties, and made me look anemic, but for this bachelorette outing with the girls, I recognized it was the only thing I already owned that would work. It would counter my lack of jewelry and makeup with a cloak of socially appropriate invisibility. I had several black pants and shirts that fit the bill, so after giving Hattie her dinner, I put on a combination of these and went to the massive living-room mirror, giving my sulky reflection some of the attention it had missed since the start of my experiment. Predictably, I found my reflection bland and dour.

Well, you wouldn't have to wear quasi yoga pants if you had a pair of decent dress jeans or black trousers, griped the Voice. *Why don't you try the leggings with the tall boots instead?*

I went to my wardrobe, put on a different all-black combination, and went back to the mirror.

Not great from behind. Try that long, dark green clingy shirt over it—it looks black. Tug it down in back. Farther. No. You could get the focus back on your face if you'd just break your stupid rules and add earrings. If you won't, then at least wear the leather jacket. Or the dress coat might deflect enough attention.

I was barely aware that I was doing all that I had sworn off in my experiment: chasing after beauty and, not ever catching it, tumbling into a morass of self-criticism and dissatisfaction. Hattie delighted in the castoffs amassing at my feet—garments, shoes, handbags—but for me, this vanity was no happy pastime. If something fit me, it went with nothing else, and if something was pretty, it was cut wrong, hemmed wrong, or stained in an obvious place. Inevitably, when I got stuck like this before a meet-up or a date, I made some bizarre last-minute choice, sweated up my blouse as I searched for my shoes, rushed out the door and forgot the keys, and then missed a train or got stuck in traffic. The evening of the bachelorette party, this panic was mounting—*No no, the belt is hideous. Take it off! Take it off!*—when John arrived home. He'd come early, so I could go out.

He slipped me a quick kiss, dropped his leaden work bag on a dining chair, and then stepped neatly in front of my reflection and plucked Hattie out of the pile of discarded clothes on the floor.

"How's this look?" I asked, hoping the nongeneric black outfit I'd cooked up would get a green light.

Openly, he looked askance. "What's that layer?" he asked. "Is that a skirt or . . . I don't know. Maybe a longer jacket?"

"It's a *tunic,*" I said, my voice brittle. "People wear them."

"Okay."

"I have to go," I said, scowling, and grabbed my not-quite-right handbag and left. Just outside, however, waiting in the mirrored lobby, was an idiot about to go public sans pants.

Changed my mind, the Voice said. *You can't do leggings.*

I stormed back inside, stripping as I went. John and Hattie scattered. I went to the closet and yanked on black blandsville. I put on a pair of black sneakers, unsuccessfully disguised as Mary Janes. I pointed to the shoes. "You know what these say?" I yelled as I tromped back past my onlookers. "They say frumpy, middle-aged stagehand!"

"What's wrong with that?" John called after me, laughing. "No one is going to see the shoes anyway! The point is to have a good time! It's your friend's party! It's supposed to be fun!"

"Yeah, lotsa fun," I yelled back and got on the elevator.

More mirrors there. Mirrors in the lobby, too. I flagged down a public minibus, climbed on, and took a window seat. My reflection was there again in the glass, crabby and unhip, a bad friend I couldn't shake.

When the bus got to my intersection, I yelled, "*Yow-lut, mgoi!*" (Stop here, please!) and jumped up, picking my way nimbly through a clutter of work bags and umbrellas. My reflection flickered in the passing windows as the bus pulled away.

"It's supposed to be fun." John's words rang in my ears as I headed down the public staircase toward the restaurant. Thanks to the matronly sneakers, I was early again. This could have been awkward, but—thanks to my experiment—I happened to know the distance between a bad mood and a good one was only a single thought. Fun. *Fun!* The extra ten minutes bought me enough time for an umbrella drink and a dogmatic commitment to good times and goodwill. When the other guests arrived, I was vivacious. When Corinne, social mastermind that she was, pulled out the pink cowboy hats, I put one on. Someone (who could it be?) started tossing penis candies onto the diners on the level below, and kissing dares were issued.

Later, we went to a dance club. As soon as you become a parent, you are forbidden to dance in public unless you are doing the hokeypokey with your child. I had my "lame and loving it" card for sure, but for a moment on the dance floor, it seemed that no one could tell. Maybe it was the devil-may-care attitude, or maybe the pink cowboy hat, or the age-inappropriate moves one can pull off in sneakers. Maybe it had just been too long since I went dancing. Whatever the reason, my uncool outfit did not inhibit my groove, but rather seemed to bring it on. When it was time to go home, there was another bonus. My feet didn't ache, nor did I long for a spandex waistband.

I walked home. Central Hong Kong's nighttime magic lies in its alleys, its tiny vinegar breweries and tea shops, its secret restaurants behind ancient doors. The cats had taken over the wetmarkets, and lovers filled the dark parklike chasms between high-rises with murmuring and playful laughter. Alongside one of the many twisting and treacherous sidewalk staircases stood a miniature shrine carefully tended by daytime hands. There were hundreds of these around the city, places where one could petition successful dead relatives or the goddesses Tin Hau and Guanyin for good luck. *Hong Kong* is the anglicized spelling of the Cantonese words *fragrant harbor,* and the city's perfume wafted out of the tiny shrine and hung in the air where I stood. Oranges and blossoms of waxy *bai eu lan* (white jade orchid) were piled in silent offering. Beside them yellow joss sticks burned slowly down to ash.

I turned to look out over my adopted city. It was glittering and dreamy through the incense smoke, but also palpably real, a mystery that unfolded around me daily. In the dark, with my reflection lost in the smoke and the Voice drowned out by the dance music still ringing in my ears, I felt more myself than I had since arriving in Hong Kong. This nighttime walker, this curious, unafraid self, this climber of dark, spooky stairs, was a beloved and familiar part of me. It was odd that I could only find her beyond the mirror like some anti-Cinderella, on the steps of a foreign city after midnight, wearing anything but fancy glass slippers.

IN EARLY MAY, I WAS OUT WITH HATTIE IN THE STROLLER WHEN WE passed a specialty paper store that sold blank, bound notebooks and unshiny ribbons in hues of "loam" and "peat." As we rolled by, I irritably noticed that the large graphic prints in the front window impeded my ability to check myself out in the glass.

I stopped. I turned us around and went back into the store. Along the rear wall, draped over wooden spindles, were large single sheets of wrapping paper in minimalist geometric and floral prints. I bought a thick stack.

When we got home, I covered the mirrors in the apartment one by one, leaving only the bathrooms free. There was not enough paper to cover every surface completely, but plenty to blot out all reflection at eye level, where it counted. When I was done, the apartment looked 50 percent smaller and darker. I'd tried to get the sheets level, but still, the walls looked messy and childish.

Uncertain about what I'd done, I made a bowl of cereal in the kitchen and came back to the dining table to eat it. I took a bite and looked up crossly, ready for validation that I was sweaty and aggravated. Pink, gray, and green squares looked serenely back at me. I shoveled in a second bite. No criticism or complaints, no reflection reminding me I should be other than I was. I was singular and anonymous in my own home.

"Hattie!" I grabbed her and tickled her with the spoon hanging out of my mouth. I stood up, tucked the bottom of my shirt into my bra, and finished my snack with my gut hanging out.

Overnight, I became a creative libertine. The day after I covered the mirrors, I rearranged the apartment: couch to the other side, bookcases moved to another room entirely, no false delineations like living room or dining room, but just the space itself as it really was, a big rectangle used for many things. The day after that, I made a sketch of a painting I wanted to do. I do not sketch or paint on a regular basis and have no talent in either, but was joyfully unimpeded by this fact. Later, I staple-gunned a couple of cork place mats together and called it a wall hanging—laughable, but recyclable. The creative effects kept coming as the week passed: Hattie got a breakfast sculpture out of kiwis and bananas, and I looked into an Ikebana flower-arranging class.

One night I did a yoga workout in our living room. Ordinarily, my reflection and I worked hard on my alignment and posture—both of which I could scrutinize in the mirrors. Now, I was compelled to listen to, and obey, the blonde contortionist on the DVD. "Open up," she commanded. "Feel something." When I did this, I felt pain. There was a soreness in my left abdomen, something, I now realized, that had been there for a while. I breathed into it, urging it to dissipate. When the DVD ended, I lay down in *savasana*, closed my eyes, and burst into tears over my dog. Two years before we left for Hong Kong, John and I had adopted a giant, aging stray off the streets. I'd had to leave Gus in the care of my parents when we moved to Hong Kong, and he'd died the week Hattie was born. The news had upset me, but I was too busy with a new infant and her unexpected heart problems to deal with my grief, so I swallowed it. I had not known it was still in there, undigested.

Something important was happening, but I wasn't sure what. My sudden spree of creativity made me think of the advice eighteenth- and nineteenth-century male artists used to get about abstaining from sex to enhance their creative powers. The idea was that by plugging one energetic leak, you could amplify the outflow elsewhere. It did feel as if I'd changed some psychic energy pattern, but the sex-creativity equation was suspicious and smacked of misogyny. Plenty of artists of both genders gathered steam from sexual topics, just as others—ahem—gathered it from neurotic self-consciousness.

More likely, I reasoned, my mirror experiment had somehow affected my "flow." I'd encountered this term while doing research on my novel that spring. Flow is a state of absorption that allows a person to do the best, hardest work she can do well: a taxi driver skillfully circumventing rush-hour traffic feels flow, as does an experienced parent deflecting a tantrum calmly, or a master chef preparing an elaborate five-course meal.* A person in flow is neither stressed nor spaced out but in the zone: unself-conscious, absorbed in her task, and often unaware of time. I always felt flow while writing, but domestic life often felt like a stretch of antiflow, rife with periods of anxious waiting (will she wake up, or can I start this task?) and peppered by mindless and frustrating disruptions. (Another goddamned hour lost to stain removal!) I knew most of this had to do with my beginner's fumbling at parenthood—but I was also fumbling so many other things at the same time. I was self-conscious about the body changes of pregnancy, as well as nervous about my roles as foreigner, not-quite-posh-enough expatriate, and dependent housewife. I might have found pleasure in the activity of learning to be who I needed and wanted to be, but I couldn't do it with a critical spectator looking over my shoulder, smashing my flow to smithereens. Covering the mirrors had temporarily blindfolded this inner critic and turned the volume of her bullying way down, allowing some portion of personal flow to return.

To my dismay, the Voice did have other channels. One rainy day, Hattie and I went down to the Bon Point mezzanine so she could practice walking. She found the reading room an excellent place to study motion, both her own, from coffee table to overstuffed chair, as well as the motion on Bonham Road, whose lively vehicular and pedestrian traffic passed one story

* Mihály Csíkszentmihályi, a founder of the positive psychology movement, is the recognized authority on this concept. It has been widely embraced across disciplines as a key to human productivity.

below the room's southern glass wall. While Hattie scrutinized red taxis and double-decker buses, I vegged. I picked up a few fashion and gossip magazines left by other residents and started flipping through. One of the magazines had an article about going a week without looking in the mirror. Child's play, I thought, puffing my own feathers. I was nearly *two* weeks into my own mirror cleanse. Next, I flipped through coverage of Elizabeth Hurley's shockingly extravagant Indian wedding in an ancient copy of *OK.*

She might have ridden in on an elephant, but she looks like cat puke by day five.

What I didn't understand about magazines like these is whether the envy, jealousy, and prurience they elicited were really mine or engineered entirely by the chatty captions. Surely, I had no ill will against Elizabeth Hurley—I didn't even know her! But I kept going, turning the page to a spread of Angelina Jolie walking with her children in New Orleans.

Hattie's way cuter than Shiloh, the Voice sniped. *Those poor kids must have such a weird life.*

I looked over to see that Hattie had worked herself into a crevasse between a baroque couch and the huge window. She was stuck, but didn't know it yet. I tried to imagine taking her to the playground with a pack of paparazzi following. They'd have a field day with us. Looking at Jolie and her kids in the magazine, I felt for them: it was one thing to have a cruel inner critic breaking your flow, but what would it be like to have outer critics doing it for you, trotting out every bad parenting moment and every low self-esteem moment and every relationship low point for the world to condemn?

They signed up for it. Celebrities know that women need somewhere else to sic the inner bitch sometimes.

Inner bitch?

I realized I wasn't vegging. Vegging was reading a book of cartoons or thumbing through a newspaper, not wildly devouring a ten-page spread on the latest celebrity debacle. What I was doing was more like sucking down half a tube of frozen Girl Scout Thin Mints. It was a binge. A binge of criticism and judgment.

"Maaaa. Maaaa!"

I slapped the magazine shut and shoved it back in the rack, carelessly ripping off a few of the front pages. I went to free Hattie from her crevasse. When we walked by the trashed magazine, she gawked at it, and at me. I'd told her all books were precious and that we must treat them with loving care. I didn't know that I'd ever said the same about people.

The habit of constant assessment was a hard one to break. Despite being well along in my mirror cleanse, I still occasionally turned to check myself out in various pieces of wrapping paper. When Anne and Eva next came over for a playdate, I asked Anne what she thought about the mirrors in *her* apartment—after all, it was nearly identical to ours.

"They're a bit much," she conceded. "But you learn to ignore it, don't you?"

I hadn't. I didn't love the look of our apartment, but I kept the wrapping paper up through April and into May.

"WE'RE MISSING THINGS," I'D SAID TO JOHN DURING THE WINTER, "and people are missing us." Hattie's babyhood was nearly over, and she still didn't recognize her grandparents. As a result, we'd planned a multicity trip back to the States in June. Travel arrangements for this trip were fraught, complex, and being handled, I felt, too exclusively by me. I was fixating on this one spring morning, as John, jet-lagged from a grueling overseas meeting, sat at the dining table. He was trying to pay bills, review credit-card statements, and sort out contradictory telecom notices in Cantonese while Hattie squirmed on his knee.

"What's this charge in Las Vegas?" he asked, looking up from a statement. "Is that the hotel room?"

"Yes, it is." Sour pause. "I asked you for input twice, but you didn't have any."

(Call my feelings about these previous one-sided interchanges a bunch of dry sticks and dead leaves that I'd been silently raking into a pile for several weeks.)

"Couldn't you get something cheaper online?" he said.

(Call this criticism a can of gasoline dumped over the pile.)

"I've been talking it over with my whole family for two weeks, and this is the decision that was made. Dad already made the reservation."

"I don't see why I have to overpay for a hotel room because you're afraid to stand up to your father."

(Call this accusation the match.)

I began to scream at John—about generosity and stinginess, about *who* was acting like a family member and who was not, about shitty time use and emotional unavailability, about helpfulness and unhelpfulness. If the mirrors had split me into two selves—one struggling to get things right and the other obsessed with detailing how I was not—uniting the two selves had unleashed a demon. I screamed to curdle milk, meaning each word to be stupefying and rank.

When I finished—probably only a minute or two later—I felt the way one feels after vomiting bile, rot, and other poisons you've brought on yourself: Spent. Also better, momentarily. But while I hadn't seen myself spitting fire, John and Hattie had witnessed the whole mess of it. Hattie, on John's knee, was paralyzed by surprise, and her eyes were as big as planets. John's face was hard. He was sitting right in front of me, but when he spoke it was as a person far away. "Do not act that way in front of our daughter again," he said.

I could say nothing. I only stood, vibrating with conflict adrenaline. I'd been intensely sure of myself while screaming, but now my family was unsure of me. For the rest of the day, I felt as if I were floating in a vacuum, a place where fear and nasty self-criticism used to rule my self-awareness, but now, it seemed, no one did.

I thought I'd regain my psychic footing when we were back in the States—surrounded by friends and family instead of covered mirrors—but that didn't happen.

Our first stop was a wedding in Los Angeles. During the reception, I told two of my closest girlfriends—both former roommates—about my experiment: laying off the hair product, skipping the jewels, and wearing the all-black stagehand's outfit I was currently suited up in.

My friend Nida, an art director with a keen eye for inconsistencies in design, listened politely as she sipped her champagne. Then she smiled broadly and said, "I can see why this is interesting, but I just don't think of you as one of those women." She shook her head, dismissive.

"You know," Amanda ventured, "this strikes me as being more about your marriage, or motherhood, or work issues than just your appearance." She fixed me with the look she uses for men who are behaving like children and said, "You *do* know you can't hide how beautiful you are."

I'd been having a lovely time at this wedding of our mutual friends, but now folded my arms across my chest and said nothing, flummoxed. I'd expected my girlfriends to be intrigued by my beauty diet, not to see through its unhappy bravado or rough me up with so much loving skepticism. I'd expected them to side with my idea, not with me.

After the wedding was the family reunion in Las Vegas. There were some nice family moments, but these were overshadowed by a gastro bug that landed Hattie in the hospital with dehydration. After that, the inner Voice sounded a lot like the emergency-room physician: *Why weren't you giving her fluids constantly and counting her wet diapers?* The answer was that I'd been worrying about family politics, worrying about John's mood, worrying that the rice was too salty for an infant and the air-conditioning too cold, and worrying that I wasn't a good-enough daughter and daughter-in-law.

In the airport lobby on our way to the East Coast, I caught sight of a rack of newspapers, all covering, ad nauseum, Paris Hilton's stint in jail. This aspect of American culture upset me; by contrast, Hong Kong's *South China Morning Post* had done a recent weekend feature on lax regulation of agricultural pesticides and rising numbers of self-poisonings by farm women. Sadly, I felt an unhappy connection between myself and the American dailies: we were both looking in the wrong direction, sweating the wrong details, fighting trivial battles when much greater injustices were at stake. I wanted to be so many things as a mother for Hattie: strong, compassionate, happy, grateful, loving, wise. Instead I was a person who screamed at her husband, who was afraid of mirrors because they reflected all her worst doubts about her own womanhood, and who—oh, yeah—sometimes forgot to keep her kid safe and healthy. I'd picked up Hattie's gastro bug but was feverish on the plane because the distance between me and the person I needed to become seemed insurmountable.

Our last stop on the trip was Long Island. We went to visit the family of a couple we'd known since college, and their grave site. They'd been driving home from a weekend in upstate New York when another driver—asleep at the wheel—crossed the freeway median and hit them head-on. Our friends had been killed instantly, and their ten-month-old daughter suffered terrible injuries, but recovered. When we visited Clara, she was eighteen months old and being cared for by an aunt. For such a visit, it was an impressively happy afternoon—the two little girls giggling and merry from start to finish. On the return bus ride, though, I held Hattie close, running my lips over her silken scalp, feeling the weight of her small body leaning into me. We had a quiet dinner and all went to bed early. Hattie climbed out of a crib we'd gone across town to borrow and got in with us.

John and I are not a couple who speak openly of what we agree on. Instead, our givens function like silent elastic tethers running between us, often running contrary to what we say and even do. These tethers remain undetectable until we've reached points too opposed. Then they yank us—sometimes roughly and fast, sometimes slowly and sweetly—back toward each other. That night grief drew us in. Our trip had been peppered with bright spots, but mostly it was dominated by illness, arguments, and logistical challenges. One of us felt it had been worth all the trouble. The other did not. As vacation trips go, it had been a hard one, and the lives we were going back to in Hong Kong held challenges for all three of us. Still, though, we had gone together through this period of time, making noise. That night, clinging to each other in the dark, we could hear it as music.

Snapshot: *Kinder Eyes*

CHATHAM, NEW JERSEY, JUNE 2011

I sit at home, on the floor, in front of my bookcase. The move to Boston is under way; boxes and packing tape are strewn around, as are my school yearbooks and photo albums. I am searching for a photo of myself taken recently, but instead I've found this other one, taken in 1994. I remember it well because my college roommates—those very roommates at the California wedding—had hung it on the door of a fridge we all shared. It made me want to cry every time I looked at it.

The photo was taken during a water-ski outing and lauded by my roommates as a "good picture." In it I am standing in a boat wearing a bright-orange life jacket, and my hair is blowing around. I am smiling. I am also twenty-five pounds heavier in the picture than I am now, pounds I fought bitterly, without success, all through high school and college. None of my roommates could understand why this picture they loved catapulted me into misery. "You look good!" they would exclaim. "You look happy!" What they could not understand was that I felt woefully misrepresented by my own body in that shot, even though I had no real evidence to this effect. I'd been overweight since puberty and chunky as a kid, with the brief exception of my few glorious months as a junior-high cheerleader.

I can't find that old cheerleading picture in this mess on my floor, either, but I remember it just as clearly: trim blue-and-white Eagles sweater, teal-blue eye shadow, shoulder-length blonde hair. I can't say my cheer picture was an accurate self-representation, either, but it did represent satisfactory achievement of an ideal. The sweater (or the eye shadow?) earned me the momentary attentions of a tall, handsome basketball player. But just as I felt the college water-skiing picture did not reflect my true self, so, too, was my true self busted in eighth grade for not living up to the sweater. The handsome ballplayer ended things after four chaste days with the self-deprecating excuse that he was not a guy who could talk to me about Shakespeare. (I knew nothing of Shakespeare in eighth grade! Nothing!)

Between the taking of the cheer picture (1988) and the taking of the water-skiing picture (1994), I read John Berger's *Ways of Seeing*. In it Berger famously says, "Men look at women. Women watch themselves being looked at." Berger also explores a split in the female self: one half of woman is the self who is constantly watched or surveyed; the other half is a cruel, internalized watcher. I did not imagine, at a boyfriendless and chubby sixteen, that by age thirty-two, I would have become a living, breathing, nit-picking example of how this bizarre female watching could tear a woman to shreds. I might have suspected it, though, because the book stayed with me through every relocation, and I have it on my shelf even now.

Although I conducted my own survey years after Berger's stewardesses-in-hot-pants seventies, our conclusions disappointingly coincide. The women in my survey thought more often about how they appeared during daily activities than the men. They also felt a far greater mismatch than men between how they looked and who they really were.

Today I manage my relationship with the mirror carefully, as well as the loud criticism it sometimes elicits. We don't live

Survey Question

Do you ever feel a mismatch between how you look and who you are?

	Women	Men
Yes	20%	9%
Sometimes	36%	39%
I used to	5%	3%
No	38%	46%

Percentage difference between how much women think about appearance during certain activities and how much men do:

Doing errands	11% more
During sex	13% more
Eating	8% more
Job or school	6% more

in a mirrored house anymore, and I've largely kicked my self-check-out habit. I don't keep fashion, beauty, or gossip magazines around because they just make me cross and yearning. Hattie hasn't seen me have a full-scale fashion meltdown in front of my reflection since that girls' night out in Hong Kong—which makes me hopeful on her behalf. Still, though, studies suggesting women and girls are fated to have a messed-up relationship to the mirror mount to the heavens.*

* According to one Oxford research summary, schoolgirls as young as six think they look fat. By age seventeen, eight out of ten girls will dislike their reflections. Women who've just tried on clothes in communal dressing rooms feel worse about what they see in the mirror, as do women who've just looked at a fashion magazine or watched a television program or ad featuring idealized female bodies and faces.

One even reported that women check their faces in the mirror an average of thirty-four times a day.

One word for this habit is *vanity.* Another is *neurosis.* Another is *perfectionism.* Another is *ambition.* Another is *hope.* The space between who we are and who we want to be can be incredibly vast for women and girls. The modern woman is an achiever, a builder, a doer, and an earner, pulling herself, her family, and sometimes her culture out of the past. Essential to this effort is an ability to doubt the merit of dear beliefs, and to ferret out one's own weaknesses. But sometimes this critical eye becomes so cold it wrecks the woman herself.

One recent afternoon, Hattie, now age five, hunkered down over two brown paper bags, a roll of tape, a pair of scissors, and a ball of twine. She waved off my snack offering and didn't look up until she had constructed and dressed herself in a full suit of armor: foot guards, shin guards, armbands, a breastplate, an apron, and a conical helmet approaching two feet in height. I helped her fasten the apron, and then she was off, a superpowered martial artist hollering and doing flying kicks from the couch.

I watched, entranced. She'd made some hats and necklaces before, but this construction was a radical departure. I hardly wanted to stop her, but raved over how amazing she looked and made her pose for a few pictures. Then I erred, grievously. "You should go check yourself out in the big mirror upstairs!" I suggested.

She did. There was silence from the bedroom, and then she stomped back down the stairs in tears, furious with me. "This hat doesn't look the way I thought it did! You said it looked good, but it doesn't! I don't like any of this!" She tore the whole amazing creation off, shredding it. Then she flung herself down on the couch, stuck her thumb in her mouth, and jammed her other hand under her armpit in a posture of babyish capitulation and self-soothing she's used since she was three months old.

"Weren't your fingers happy making the armor?" I asked Hattie, going over and rubbing her back. "Wasn't your body happy jumping off the couch?"

I kissed and consoled her because I understood her dilemma: it's hard to get the real world to match our imagination of it, and sometimes it never does.

In these moments, perhaps the best choice is to turn away from the mirror and rely on those eyes that see us through a rose-colored lens of love. These are the eyes that see the beauty of happiness in all our "fat" pictures and see the anxiety of a hard breakup through lost pounds and new clothes. These eyes can tell the difference between a strict new program of self-correction and a longer journey of true self-acceptance. They see our giant paper-bag helmet as an awesome example of ingenuity, not a silly hat. A suave male admirer once told me that beautiful women never get to see themselves dancing.

Here it is. Now I've got it, this picture I was looking for, dug up in a desk drawer, not the bookshelf at all. It was taken while Hattie and I were on our first major mother-daughter adventure together—a long drive, a hotel stay, an unfamiliar city. I didn't think much of this shot at first, but I am beginning to trust it. In it I am sitting on a sunny porch, eating breakfast earlier than I would have liked. My hair is freaking out to one side, and I'm smiling. I look, somewhat unbelievably, young, strong, sure, and happy.

Hattie took it.

In the picture I am holding a teacup, but what I see is a woman dancing.

6

Itsy Bitsy Teeny-Weeny Fertility Advertisement

A man has every season while a woman only has the right to spring.

—JANE FONDA, ACTRESS, FORMER FASHION MODEL, FITNESS GURU, AND POLITICAL ACTIVIST

HONG KONG AND MALAYSIAN SABAH, JULY 2007

One summer morning, about five months into the experiment, Hattie and I went to the apartment-complex pool, and my bathing suit decomposed. It was already nearly transparent in spots; now the elastic ceded defeat by chlorine as well. I had to hold it in place with one hand while we bobbed to prevent it from peeling down like a banana skin. I'd been feeling pretty good that a jungle at my bikini line and braidable armpits didn't stop me from taking Hattie for a dip, but this was different. I was now approaching nudity poolside. The situation was dire enough that when I walked past a swimwear shop in Central the next day, I went in. I saw a possibility on the first rack, took it into the dressing room, and stripped.

Something unusual happened. I did not hear *Zikes* or *Try again.* Instead, I heard *Okay. Now turn around.* When I turned, I didn't see a rear profile of four separate buttocks (two swinging free outside the sausage casing, two jam-packed inside), nor did my boobs float around like jellyfish in a sandwich bag or fall out when I bent over. I reeled with disbelief, flashing back to the million hours I'd spent schlepping in and out of dressing rooms, griping to girlfriends about how wide or skinny or fat or thin my whichever body part was and how no bathing suit on the planet was ever cut to flatter. But now, in this single convergence of circumstance, timing, and retail geography, the unthinkable had happened in less than ten minutes: I loved the very first suit I tried on, and it fit. Fate, perhaps—or was my experiment having a positive effect?

Either way, I bought the suit, wincing at my treachery and the price (seventy dollars). I had fallen off my experimental wagon, hard. But was there any woman I knew who would not have done the same when needing a bathing suit and encountering this once-in-a-lifetime magical swimwear scenario—even if she'd made vows of shopping abstinence a few months earlier? I could come up with no one.

Later that night, I dutifully dropped an equivalent wad of cash in my philanthropy jar. It was a sorry pot, because once I'd stopped shopping for real, I lost interest in the activity of judging goods for pleasure. I just didn't want to go into stores and experience all that mania. The downside was that I wasn't dropping in much money for a wished-for pair of flats here or an alluring tube of face cream there. It bothered me that my plan was not working out as I'd imagined it, but my recent backsliding suggested that I should keep skipping the stores. My delight in my new two-piece bathing suit was tainted by guilt, but still very much there. It was better than a two-piece, actually. It was a bikini.

Frenchman Louis Reard cooked up the modern bikini in 1946 expressly to showcase women's youth and fertility. He probably didn't think of it that way, but the bikini does what no other garment can: advertise a woman's hourglass figure, something that signals fertility in a number of ways. Hip fat means fetus-friendly nutritional resources and hormonal balance in a woman, whereas waist fat, among other liabilities, signals age and menopause. From zaftig Marilyn to skinny Kate Moss, nearly every woman deemed physically beautiful conforms to what has been called the golden ratio and as a consequence looks great in a bikini.* For all the rest of us out there, a well-cut bikini can make a less-than-ideal waist-hip ratio look a lot better.

I took my little black fertility advertisement along with us when we headed to Malaysian Sabah for a long weekend in late July. This was a real vacation for all of us, no family obligations, no emergency room or projectile vomiting, just a hotel on a jungly beach in Borneo. The bay there was windswept, well protected, and nearly empty. It was hard not to feel a back-to-the-Garden innocence when walking along it without very much on. In my new bikini, I could imagine myself wild and free and miles beyond the reach of sunless tanner, miracle

* A woman with this golden ratio has a waist eight-tenths the width of her hips or less. Brain researcher and psychologist Nancy Etcoff compiles several studies in which researchers measured the waist-hip ratio of beautiful women in a range of eras. As it turns out, Miss Americas from the twenties, *Playboy* models in the fifties, *Playboy* models in the nineties, supermodels, fashion models, and glamour models all hit that golden ratio of .8 or below. Most are below it—meaning even curvier—becoming what Etcoff calls "sex-bombs" as they approach Barbie's physiologically impossible but instinctively alluring waist-hip differential of .54.

suits, cellulite creams, and expensive depilation. Hattie thrilled at the roll and suck of the gentle waves while she clung to me and then waddled ashore and scrubbed at the clean sand with her feet. It calmed me to do as she did: gaze for long minutes at the bobbling yellow sea kayaks and the improbable ascent of the parasailer under a rainbow chute.

It was while in this blissfully refreshed state of mind one afternoon that I gathered our towels and herded Hattie back toward the rooms for a nap. John was already taking one, and I thought I might join him. We ambled past an outdoor bar, a table-tennis cabana, and, next to it on the sand, a volleyball court. A few guests were hitting the ball around. As Hattie paused to inspect something in the sand, I spotted a young woman in a black bikini like mine, facing away.

Look at this, hissed the Voice.

Reflexively, I scanned the girl from top to bottom and back up again. I took in the unbound dark hair that reached to her shoulder blades, the lean arms without an ounce of wiggle underneath, the slender waist, and those two small curved marks of loveliness on her lower back above an impossibly cellulite-free rear end.

You'll never have that.

I took in her long legs as she lunged for the ball, tossed her hair, and laughed. My eyes narrowed, and the back of my neck prickled as I wondered how she could be *so lean,* and yet . . . nothing about her was bony or pinched. She was undeniably feminine: a nymph with the sort of body that tossed all my best efforts at eating sensibly and exercising regularly in my face. If I had a tail, I'd have swished it.

And then she turned, called out "Mama!" and ran to embrace a middle-aged woman exiting the hotel. I drew in my claws as my heart sank with shame. The object of my envy was thirteen. Maybe fourteen. When she turned her pretty face, it was so obviously a child's: clear, sweet, and still dear to her parents in the very way Hattie's face was dear to me and John. The poor kid had done nothing to me except exist at that cusp of girlhood when parents begin to sweat about hemlines and rage about bared midriffs and lipstick. But in her tiny black bathing suit, the promise of her womanhood was on display: to the male bartenders, volleyball players, and hotel guests. And so was the present reality of mine—no longer young, not ever as pretty, less a fertile woman in a bikini than a human coat rack with an assortment of damp towels, discarded sand toys, and an "I'm busy" sign hanging off me.

Chastened and depressed, I scooped up my junior excavator in her sandy diaper, settled her comfortably on my pooch belly, and started back toward our room. Why, I wondered, was my instinct to compete with this girl's beauty instead of celebrating it? And why, when I was her age, had I never felt as beautiful and powerful as I must have been?

One of the advantages of being a heterosexual female over twenty-five is that you know your male partner is *not* going to understand or be empathetic about your appearance angst. Also, the mood will pass or, better yet, be interrupted. As Hattie and I entered our room, we heard panicky yelping and crashing from the bathroom. John was being terrorized by a four-inch cockroach.

I took the rubber sandal from his hand and stepped in boldly, casting my shadow upon that vermin and showing it my experienced face of doom. It buzzled and zipped behind the wastebasket; I lunged and stomped, my pooch belly heaving and my underarms waggling as John and Hattie cheered me on. Eventually I pulverized that crunchy disease vector, landing hits no scrawny teenager could have matched.

It was not during these bathroom high jinks but afterward—when John had deftly shushed Hattie into a nap and we were lying on the bed sharing a victory Shasta—that I began to feel my funk start to break up. If I was not a bikini babe sitting on the cover of *Sports Illustrated*'s swimsuit issue, I reasoned, then neither was John that bare-chested mechanic stud holding the two tires. At present, he was comically piebald from badly applied sunscreen, uncommonly happy and relaxed, and watching wacky Malaysian television with me. If the biological function of beauty was to stop the opposite sex in their tracks, then hey, we'd done it—to each other. And now

Survey Questions

What, if anything, has ever caused your definition of "sexually attractive" to change, shift, or expand?

	Women	Men
Age	52%	46%
Person	39%	39%
Relationship	43%	30%
My looks	19%	7%
Other	15%	10%
No change	8%	14%

In what state do you think your current or most recent relationship partner finds you sexiest?

	Women	Men
Home or casual look	38%	39%
Totally au natural	23%	18%
Dressed for work	19%	22%
Decked out	19%	19%

the man I was lying next to was less a man-on-the-make than a man-holding-the-remote, a separate species entirely, one I had come to love for so many reasons beyond the broad shoulders, cellist's sculpted forearms, and deep voice that had first turned me on.

The shape of sexual attraction was bound to evolve, I reasoned, like everything else, especially between two people in love for a long time. The evidence? Despite the difficulty of managing it in a hotel room with a crib shrouded in beach towels not three feet away—John and I managed to do, that afternoon, what couples often do on vacation.

I WOULD BE LYING IF I SAID THAT I DIDN'T GIVE BIKINI BABE another thought. I stayed on high alert the remainder of the trip, possibly because this is the nature of a beach resort where people walk around in bathing suits all day. But the Malaysian state of Sabah is largely Muslim, and when we left the hotel, the rules changed. The young women at the markets and tourist attractions we visited were in loose traditional blouses and sarongs or in jeans, long sleeves, a *hijab,* and closed-toe shoes.

This ubiquitous public modesty put my own Western dressing habits in sharp perspective. When we went to see a dance performance, my tank top and Western shorts felt immodest and tarty as I sat down among a crowd of local Sabans, and the skin of my upper arms and thighs offensively overexposed. As we waited for the show to start, I remembered one morning early in my experiment when I'd been dazzled by the graceful way a young woman had carried herself as she crossed a street. I'd noticed her dancer's posture because she'd been dressed in baggy, unattractive clothes with her hair in a floppy ponytail. Now I recognized that if that dancer had been wearing a miniskirt and heeled boots, or even showing as much skin as I was showing right now at the show, the whole positive chain reaction would have been sabotaged. My nasty, sexually competitive inner Voice would have whispered *Bitch.* Quickly, I picked Hattie up and set her on my lap; as an attention deflector, she rarely failed,* and warm smiles from fellow audience members quickly followed.

As John, Hattie, and I went on that day to browse through a local Saban market—all the vendors more modestly concealed than I was—I wondered whether some enterprising female researcher had ever found an increase in female cooperation and goodwill in societies that banned sexy advertisements and enforced (weather-appropriate) modesty or even uniforms. I sort of hoped she had. In the next second, I hoped she hadn't—or wouldn't—until I was fifty and had clearly lost the upper hand.

Because I couldn't decide whether I was for liberated exposure of the female body or for cooperative concealment, I did some directed people watching in the airports on our way back to Hong Kong. Clearly, the world's women had not gotten the memo about staying on message with their bodies and clothes; the variety of information they sent about wealth, age, culture, marital status, and religion was staggering: Western shorts and tank tops could bare tantalizing youthful limbs, but they also broadcast aggressive mature concern for comfort

* She almost failed dangerously, once. In Singapore, I'd knelt facing into the corner of a shady public building to breast-feed her. As we left, we passed tourists being cloaked in long robes and head coverings by stern handlers. I'd accidentally bared my breasts in a mosque and done it in a country where walking around naked in your own house could get you arrested.

over local custom. *Salwar kameez* concealed youthful South Asian figures, whereas saris exposed ample maternal midriffs in swaths of gold-edged fabric. Muslim caftans and head scarves piously concealed the female shape but sometimes revealed thickly made-up faces and bloodred toenails in jeweled sandals. Then, when we deplaned into the billboard-rich environment of the Hong Kong International Airport, I encountered an array of female bosoms, legs, and shoulders suggesting I buy things. If I did, my own body would become free advertising space for the brands. This system was gangbusters in label-crazy Hong Kong—no one seemed the slightest bit embarrassed to be a walking mannequin.

After John, Hattie, and I retrieved our luggage, we boarded the Airport Express train for the trip back to Central. I was looking forward to a quick nap, but there in the miniature seat-back screen, a young woman was conveying an earnest message about the great work the Chinese government was doing to clean up a recent mining cave-in. Although she was fully clothed, she reminded me of the young female models I saw portrayed in the art galleries along Hollywood Road: nude or mostly nude, they positioned bare sections of themselves prettily among pencils and erasers or stood in the snow, holding assault rifles. They were oddly generic, these lean, long-haired females between seventeen and thirty, as if they weren't different women but the same woman-pictograph used over and over, always softening someone else's artistic, commercial, or political agenda.*

* There are female artists who've claimed their bodies as their own canvases. To name a few: in 1965 Yoko Ono allowed an audience to cut off her clothes, in 1969 Valie Export offended public modesty by walking around in crotchless pants, in 1972 Eleanor Antin photographed herself wasting away on a crash diet, in 1975 Carolee Schneeman pulled a long letter about creativity out of her vagina, and in 2009 Kate O'Brian and Sinead King, a.k.a. "The Muffia," flashed fake pubic hair at passersby outside department stores.

The irony was that many young, beautiful, and fertile women in Hong Kong were sending an entirely different message with their bodies. Hong Kong's public radio station had recently done a story on the problem of Mainland Chinese women entering Hong Kong as the mistresses of residents and then refusing to leave. Pregnant Mainlanders would wait until labor had started and then give birth "accidentally" in a Hong Kong hospital. And the Airport Express train we were currently on passed close to Tin Shui Wai, a remote, industryless housing block familiarly known as the "City of Sadness." I couldn't see the buildings from the train, but this warehouse of poverty had become notorious earlier in the spring, when one crazed young mother threw her two children, and then herself, out a fifty-story window. Authorities later admitted she was not the first destitute woman to do so. It wasn't being painted or pinned up on billboards, but this was a message from the female body, too: the ultimate protest.

My own life had almost nothing in common with that woman's troubled one, yet I felt in one way connected to her—and to the modest Sabans, the dancer with perfect posture, even the models in paintings and on billboards, and the pretty teenager at the beach. Our female bodies, the public promise of their fertility, and the children they did or did not produce would, in many ways, define our lives. As I looked out at the brilliant green hills of grass speeding by, I tried to imagine a world in which every female body sent healthy, satisfied messages about this truth of womanhood, messages that were more often positive than painful.

I couldn't quite imagine that world, but I wanted to.

TOWARD THE VERY END OF MY EXPERIMENT, NEARLY SIX MONTHS after that trip to Malaysia, I gained a final perspective on the problem—and promise—of the female body as an advertising medium. My friend Petra invited me to a girls' night out organized by her Russian club, and I accepted. This wasn't just any old dinner and drinks; it was a dance class, a *lap-dancing* class. By then I wasn't as hesitant as I might have been earlier in the year—what could embarrass me more than I'd already embarrassed myself? I was also curious about what I'd first noticed living in San Francisco: the woman-driven sexpot renaissance: boudoir photography, recreational stripping, trashy adult Halloween costumes. Maybe the best way to own the message one's own body sent was to beef up its sexual allure, that is, learn to outfox any pretty sixteen-year-old in a bikini and then walk through the world knowing it.

The class was not held in a well-lit yoga or fitness studio, as it might have been in the United States. Instead, it was downhill from our apartment in the dim quarters where abalone were dried and warehoused during the day and where no one seemed to be at eight o'clock on a weeknight. I saw my friend Petra outside the address, and she pulled me into a tiny, crowded elevator filled with high-decibel Russian giggles. The elevator rose, grinding ominously under our combined weight, and then released us into a room kitted out like a dance studio, except it had poles.

Poles! Right away, all of us started swinging, climbing, and hanging. Who cared if we were more simian than sexpot; the poles were so much fun! Money was collected, clothes were shed, high heels were strapped on. We'd been told to bring them, to get in the right mood.

Our Australian instructor was older than I expected but had big hair and was dressed in short-shorts. She had a perfect waist-hip ratio but was no clothes hanger.

"I have two kids, and I live with my husband," she started, "and this class is about feeling good about yourself and your body. It's about expressing yourself sexually."

Murmuring and giggles all around. The instructor cranked up a mix of my least-favorite classic rock and led us through an exercise in self-stroking, hair tossing, and slinking around the room. I went through the motions, loosening my pelvis while worrying about my black-bean lunch; nothing like farting to kill a mood. Then we addressed the dance.

"The first thing you should understand," the instructor said, "is that you are always in control of what is happening." She went on to demonstrate how to position a man in a chair so we could get away, so that whatever happened was what we wanted to have happen. "This is something you choose to do," she admonished. "It's your show."

But it wasn't our show, yet. If it had been, we would have been facing the mirrors or, better yet, blindfolded, concentrating on how the dancing felt. Instead, we each faced our own empty folding chair, while our instructor taught us how to "rock around the clock" and do the crotch crunch and advised us never, ever, if we were facing away from our victim and leaning over, to peek between our legs.

"See what happens?" she said, all red-faced and mashed up. "Not sexy."

Another tip was this: "If you really want a man to pay attention, come into the room, strike a pose, and then drop to your knees and crawl."

So much for being in control.

The class *was* fun, no doubt about it. Part of what made it fun was that it was harder than it looked. I tried out my skills on John shortly thereafter, who was mildly impressed. Any sizzle I'd evoked petered out, though, when Hattie woke up mid-dance and had to be tended. That killed my stripper's buzz, and as I rocked and hushed, I wondered when—if ever—it would be *my* turn to sit on the couch with a martini and be wowed. It's said that women control the household finances; maybe these classes would do even better if they were designed for couples.*

Again, hard to imagine. But trying to helped me think maybe I'd been looking at physical beauty—the beauty messages of my own body, especially—from the wrong, red-faced, upside-down angle.

Snapshot: *Measurements*

Boston, July 2011

Suddenly, we live in Boston, smack in the middle of downtown. It's a temporary apartment, way up on the thirty-second floor. The views are reminiscent of Hong Kong, as is the street culture: narrow bricked alleys, pristine public parks, bookstores, a

* A cultural anthropologist shared this observation with me: Pornography consumption on campuses is changing because women can now access porn privately and anonymously on the Internet. While this can lead to butterfly Brazilians and "designer vaginas" in sexually active young women, it also gives these women considerable performance expectations of their sexual partners. It's hard to imagine a man showing off his fake orgasm over a pastrami sandwich the way Meg Ryan did in *When Harry Met Sally*, but it seems that young men are becoming more self-conscious and body-conscious during sex, so we may be headed in that direction.

waterfront. I feel invigorated by everything around us, but I also feel terribly old when I plow, with my double stroller, through the young professionals walking to offices in trendy dresses and the teenagers sitting on the grassy Boston Common. The suburbs—with their high concentration of middle-aged parents—seem to have lessened the blow of age, while the city emphasizes it.

Age is the bitterest vitamin. What was an unpleasant but manageable taste during my experiment has got me in a full pucker four years later: there are sharp lines around my mouth now and a sprinkle of wiry silver hairs where there once sprang a pluckable one. It's hard to believe, as everything begins to soften and drape, that this can possibly be good and that I can wrest an ounce of happiness from such obviously fading beauty. The occasional sensation of over-and-doneness is amplified when I think of our family situation. We've already been blessed with two children, so what does this mean for all this used reproductive equipment I've got hanging around? In a rare moment of desperation over this, I stoop to asking John for a direct compliment on my body.

"It can be anything," I tell him. "Maybe my ankles, or my retinas."

"You keep saying you need a new bathing suit," he says, "but you look good in your black one. You have a cute butt."

Holy frijoles. Score another point for the black bikini. Even though I'd fished for this compliment, I am shocked, flattered, and more than anything reminded that although I might feel eighty-seven years old sometimes, I am only thirty-six and John is the same, and between us we have 350 million years of road-tested sexual and genetic advertising that has successfully filled the planet with human beings.

Since my experiment, I've looked to science for help parsing the power of the bikini babe, and it's remarkably simple.

All you need is the big three: an hourglass figure, facial beauty, and youth. And just as an hourglass figure is an actual mathematical ratio, so are these other requirements strictly defined. Any woman of any race in the world judged to be attractive by men, women, children, and infants as young as three months will likely have a symmetrical face with fairly average features that conform to the basic human face plan for females: small chin and jaw; large, widely-spaced eyes; high cheekbones; and full lips.* The definition of youth is even simpler and more direct: it means nulliparous, or having never given birth. Yesterday's Man, supposedly, discovered that the best way to ensure a woman carried his seed was to nab a virgin. Teenagers were judged the best genetic investment, a perception that is possibly responsible for the facts that most supermodels are signed in their early teens and most brides in traditional cultures are between the ages of twelve and fifteen.

Sigh. According to evolutionary biology, there is no help for women—we're either too young to know what we have or too old to have it anymore. But as I age, I'm not so willing to shrug this off. Modern fertility science is now undermining the reliability of the big-three signals.† Most of us frown on adults

* Here's why science likes these features: body symmetry means a fetus developed properly in the womb, and average features are safer for organisms to have than outstanding ones. (For example, birds with unusually long wingspans might fly faster or higher than others when winds are calm, but are more often killed in storms.) As for the basic human face plan, it reflects normal hormonal balance and an absence of deformity or other genetic abnormality. Supermodels—upon whose looks people often disagree—often have features that *exaggerate* nature's favored, averaged proportions. So, while widely spaced eyes may be universally attractive in a woman, a supermodel may have eyes as widely spaced as a toddler, or she may have unusually full lips. If she has both, or if any single feature is too exaggerated, she may cross the line into unattractive or simply weird.

† Sometimes the hot bikini babe is on the Pill, sometimes the fertile woman is a surrogate, and sometimes the smoothest skin may be indicative of a budget for plastic surgery, not youth.

marrying teens, eat delicious donuts instead of nutritious grubs, and, for the most part, are not interested in having ten children and do what we must to keep those numbers down. Also, that evo-bio assessment of why men get hot for women has some detractors in the scientific community. Love, they say, might be as profitable a genetic investment as youth, which makes sense when you think about how many humans have *siblings*. Most important of all, the life of a modern woman in a developed nation is not exclusively defined by her cycles of fertility. Chances are good she'll live forty years past her peak bikini days—far too long to spend mourning their passing or trying to get them back.

Still, the imperfect or aging female body is a sore spot for women—one that most men don't seem to share. Here, in Boston, I recently spoke with a woman in her seventies who complained that her elderly female friends would not come to cool off in her lovely backyard pool because they did not want to be seen, even by each other, in bathing suits. I've had friends of mine declare themselves too old for bikinis because they felt pregnancy-softened waists, hips, and breasts had become liabilities. My own passing years make me more compassionate about all the things women do to try to retain bikini babeness. It's easy to dismiss the bone-crushing corsets and rocket bras of yesterday, but harder to wave off Spanx and Not-Your-Daughter's jeans once you've given birth; harder to shun the mystical, chemical promises of Retinol and La Mer once you've hit thirty-five; harder, once you've realized that sun damage is permanent, to turn your nose up at those minimally invasive surgeries that promise to make the outside look as young as the inside feels. When I look at my own deepening dimples and softening neckline, I sometimes doubt I can cultivate enough charms to make up for the lost attractiveness of youth. And when I start to worry too much about this, I think of two very different women—the first one, my mother.

When I was a kid, I believed most of Mom's criticisms about herself—that she had a weak profile, shoulders that did not hold straps well, and a belly that tended to get "potty." It was a surprise to me, as a teenager, to find Mom intensely beautiful one day as we were working in our garden in Vermont. She was telling me something, the loam dropping off her trowel, but I heard none of what she said. I saw only the light in her hazel eyes and the vitality of the skin along her collarbones. She'd rolled up the sleeves of her turquoise T-shirt, exposing lean, tanned arms. My mother's mature, adult beauty was a revelation to me, when I finally recognized it. She was in her forties by then, had triumphed over years of depression, and was beginning to reconnect with an artistic aptitude that she'd abandoned before my brother and I were born. She was also working very hard on herself, not on the shape of her hips and breasts, but on the contours of her own life, and the life she shared with my father.

Today, at sixty-five, Mom's paintings hang in galleries around the Southwest. She and my dad are still married, but she sometimes travels independently, sometimes tells him off, regularly eats food he won't touch, and can swim a mile. Last spring I saw her a few moments after a workout and, again, found her gorgeous, even in a bathing suit she calls a "baggy old thing" and with her wet hair slicked perfectly flat. She might not have had the waist-hip ratio of an eighteen-year-old, but she had the radiance of someone whose body and the life it gives are cherished. At sixty-five, my mom is the antidote to all those pretty teenagers I was struggling with during my experiment—a bikini babe who's realized the value of her female body didn't end with her youth.

If Ma can do it, I figure, so can I. A few days after I ask John for my compliment, I slip out the apartment door at dawn for a jog. When I sprint across a rusty, old train bridge, I feel my arms, legs, and abs waking up, getting ready to carry me through rich decades of womanhood that I know not every woman in the world is lucky enough to have.

The second woman I think of, when my age or waning fertility starts to get me down, is that desperate young mother who will never appear on billboards or in painted portraits, the one without measurements, now defined only by her absence. I sometimes imagine that my own heart caught her, and her children, in midair and that her body's message of pain was printed there to speed me, and all of us, toward a better future.

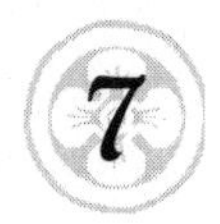

The Professionals

> Look like a girl, act like a lady, think like a man and work like a dog.
>
> —Caroline K. Simon, lawyer, New York secretary of state, adviser to the UN, judge

Hong Kong, August 2007

It was at *yum cha* that I spoke with my beauty nemesis, Aubrey Cook, for the first time. *Yum cha,* or Chinese brunch, is one of the great Hong Kong traditions: you sit, you gab, you drink jasmine tea and eat cholesterol-soaked morsels too elaborate to prepare at home. Only a few months into my experiment, and my friend Ruth had corralled a number of young families to meet up at Jumbo, a famous floating restaurant in Aberdeen Harbor. Its five stories of wood, lights, balconies, and lanterns had crumbled in the late 1980s, but it was now restored to original Hollywood-ish glamour.

Touristy though it was, and not known for superior cuisine, it was still a treat to take the short boat ride across the harbor and step out onto red carpet flanked by green marble lions.

Since I'd been briefly introduced to Aubrey at Ruth's house once before (back when I was still wearing dangly earrings to playdates), I chose a seat next to her and began fussing over Hattie's high chair. If Aubrey remembered me, she didn't acknowledge it. She tossed her dark-blonde ponytail over her shoulder, leaned away from me, and started pouring tea for everyone. Ruth handed around menus, orders and introductions were made, and the food arrived.

It was between the spare ribs and the razor clams that I noticed Aubrey and I, as well as our two husbands, weren't having the luck that people getting to know each other sometimes have. Instead, we slogged through unending context: Where exactly in the United States were we from, and which company was John working with? Where had we gone to school? We were both asking and both answering, but somehow the exchange of words never warmed into conversation. I also had the feeling that Aubrey was closely assessing me, and consequently I fumbled my chopsticks, smacked my lips, and very nearly spat a bone straight onto my plate, a move that is perfectly acceptable at a Chinese table, but iffy among expats. But it's not so unusual to miss a connection in a noisy restaurant while holding a child down in a high chair she doesn't like. When we parted ways after the outing, I'd considered our interchange neutral, our relationship unformed, possibly never to form.

A few weeks later, though, I ran into Aubrey at the supermarket.

"Hello, Phoebe. How are you." The ice in Aubrey's voice froze any possible reply in my mouth. She gave me a quick scan—the same down-up-down I'd used on the bikini girl in Borneo—and then she walked past me and away. I had never been openly addressed with such disdain. I spent the rest of the day thawing out, perplexed.

First, I wondered if I'd offended Aubrey somehow at the brunch. I could come up with nothing. Then I wondered if I was simply "not the sort of person" Aubrey wanted to hang with in Hong Kong. I did not belong to a club, had been ignorant of the important preschool waiting lists, and, along with John, possibly presented a messier social package than Aubrey was used to encountering in her smallish island nation. Maybe she did not have a working set of etiquette rules for our multiculti, mixed-grill sort of union. But this old-school *Us versus Them* objection seemed too dated in the context of postcolonial Hong Kong. The city today is a teeming cultural mash-up, a point surely not lost on Aubrey, self-avowed lover of travel.

But if Hong Kong is a mixed bag of mixed bags, expatriate Hong Kong can also feel like a small town where you run into your least-favorite neighbor again and again. I next saw Aubrey at Ruth's, up in the gardens at the Peak, and in the bookshop. We should have had plenty to talk about, but unless Ruth was there, it was always unmitigated ice.

I mused, I mulled, I scolded myself that my experiment made me a victim of heightened self-consciousness and a nutcase. Nevertheless, I could not avoid my dawning conviction that Aubrey Cook didn't like me because I looked so freaking bad. And I did: by late summer, the Sun-In-lightened streaks in my hair had grown out, my summer wardrobe looked as old as it was, and I was approaching something I'd never before achieved: equivalent prep time. John's morning routine took him about twelve minutes, and by middle August, mine was down to sixteen: shower, comb hair, apply deodorant, slather

SPF 30 moisturizer on all exposed skin, dress, done.* But could a person really hate me for a crappy haircut and grungy sandals? It began to seem possible.

Aubrey herself was neither homely nor stunning but blessed, as most of us are, with strengths to counteract weaknesses: a smooth brow and pale-gold irises turned the gaze from largish feet. But what truly set Aubrey apart was her impeccable grooming. During *yum cha,* in the grocery, out for a walk, probably in bed, and possibly even while sitting on the toilet, Aubrey was always perfectly event appropriate and enhanced with jewelry and makeup calibrated to the hour—nay, *demi*hour—of the day. This is not to say she overdid it—she would no more wear Juliet's red death-scene dress to her husband's work party than slacks to a barbecue. But she did seem to achieve the Catalog Ideal of herself, daily. When I spotted her in the grocery, she was dressed in updated classics with a smattering of trendy items, sporting a hairstyle that was meant to look practical but was actually loose and romantic, carrying a baguette and leafy greens in her basket beside a bar of soap that matched her shoes. She inflicted this precision on her kid, too. I never saw the child in anything less than eye-popping cuteness, all unstained clothes in the right size.

Now, most of the women I hung out with during my experiment—Anne and Grace or my Friday-afternoon crew—had nice clothes in a range of styles and certainly paid more attention to their grooming than I did. If these friends noticed my unkempt state, they seemed to chalk it up to a quirk of personality, lack of interest, or bad shopping tech-

* For everyone counting, I waited until after breakfast to brush my teeth.

nique. My "look" was only one of a number of qualities that cemented a relationship, and in other realms I was at least holding my own. With Aubrey, whenever I came within thirty feet of her, my inner Voice channeled a barrage of (imagined?) internal criticism from her: "God, running shoes with a skirt? No makeup *at all—ever?* That terrible, terrible haircut without a single blonde streak? No earrings? Why, why, *why* the stained top? The badly or unwaxed legs? The lack of toenail polish? And what the hell is the story with those godawful shoes?" (The story was that my podiatrist had diagnosed swollen ligaments in my left foot and condemned me to closed-toe shoes and orthotics indefinitely. I tried to honor this grim prescription, but sometimes rebelled with a pair of broken-down flat sandals. Once upon a time they had been canvas colored and "unusual." Now they were dirt colored, the treads filled with fossilized gum. They also now missed the metal studding that set them apart and had an organized pattern of holes instead.)

I recognized the possibility that I was just projecting all this animosity from Aubrey, but when I mentioned the static between us to John one spring evening (we were draping damp laundry around the apartment), he didn't say, "Oh, come on. It's all in your mind," as I was expecting. Instead, he paused with a white undershirt in his hand and said thoughtfully, "Yeah. She's tough."

I was floored. John's saying "She's tough" was equivalent to a girlfriend's saying "That woman is a total bitch." Whether Aubrey was or wasn't, John's response confirmed for me that the static I felt was real.

OVER THE SUMMER, AUBREY INVITED US TO HER DAUGHTER'S birthday party. When I discovered the pretty blue-and-green envelope in our mailbox, I immediately understood this was a natural extension of Aubrey's public persona. She was good and gracious to invite everyone; some of us would wisely decline. And I'd meant to decline, too, except Ruth didn't let me.

"I know she can be a pill," Ruth whispered to me with the exasperated abandon of the nine-months pregnant. "Just go to see her place. She *loves* having guests."

By coincidence, John's colleague was also hosting a party later that same day on the same side of the island. It was too hot for Hattie to play outside for long, and if we timed it right, we wouldn't have to think about lunch or dinner. We decided to attend both.

On the designated day, my concessions to party format were thus: I brought a nice present for the birthday girl, and all of us were germ free, bathed, and dressed in clothes without obvious holes or stains (with the exception of my shoes, which I knew would be abandoned at the door), and we arrived on time.

Our hostess herself answered the door, dressed in gilded lace and perfect jeans.

"Phoebe. Hello," Aubrey said, her eyebrows trying to climb her face in dismay, but being held down by hostessing willpower. I had RSVP'd; she'd probably blocked it out. She stepped back a smidgen and rested her fingertips on the sideboard behind her—the better to administer a laser-powered once-over as we tumbled in over the pile of strollers and diaper bags. It didn't matter that I had spent almost six months nurturing confidence in my honest, unaltered appearance. In six seconds, Aubrey eviscerated it. Half-moons burned under my eyes where concealer should have been.

"You know, Ruth's had the baby," Aubrey told me.

"I got a text," I said, "but no details."

"I stopped by the hospital this morning," Aubrey said. "After my swim." Aubrey was training for a charity triathlon. "They're doing quite well," she went on. "You should go up and see her."

"I should. I know."

There was a grim pause during which I noticed Aubrey's diamond earrings and she noticed my sandals of the living dead. She and I both looked at Hattie, whose finger was up her nose to the second knuckle. Half of John's shirt was tucked in, the other half not.

"Aubrey, you remember my husband, John," I said.

"Yes, *hello*, John," she said, her disinterest infinite. "So good to see you again." A sharklike blankness deepened those gold irises, but she fabricated a smile and ushered us inside. "Olivia!" she barked to another new arrival, and we were dismissed.

John and I wandered into a hall lit like a museum. It was hung with original pencil sketches and had weavings—not rugs—on the floor. We passed a cluster of women in big necklaces and exited into a living room straight out of *Architectural Digest*. John spotted the snack table piled high with the delicacies I sampled in the grocery but never bought, and he peeled off. In an effort to look less aimless and friendless than I was, I sat down on the floor with Hattie and covertly looked around.

Aubrey's home felt not like a residence, but like a Disneyland for grown women of good taste. There were walnut end tables, specialty lighting fixtures, those pod footrest things from Turkey, and draperies that matched them and fell just so. There were art books, tall vases, and actual sculpture. The few toys littering the floor looked like the droppings of a guilty rainbow dog. I wondered briefly if this domestic perfection was just one of those "company's coming" cleanup jobs, but a person couldn't just hunt down a set of antelope horns or plant a rooftop butterfly garden in the two hours before a party. Aubrey had only been in Hong Kong as long as we had, and even with a toddler in tow, she'd managed this?

I stayed put for longer than I should have, watching the babies play on the sunny rug. But I was also eavesdropping on the shopping talk of two women sitting on the couch near me (new department store again) and then eavesdropping on Aubrey as she chatted animatedly with another female guest. The guest was crooning over the apartment's loveliness, but Aubrey was dismissive. Her real interest was back home in the house she and Philippe were designing from the ground up. Aubrey's conversation partner looked appropriately awed. They moved on to the artwork now, and as I wrestled a shape sorter out of the toy basket, I heard Aubrey speak, as I'd never heard her speak, of her past career as a buyer for a large department store. Later she'd become an exec in public relations and marketing.

Ding. The not-so-special light fixture in my own brain went on. Aubrey didn't achieve Catalog Idealism because she was a dabbler or hobbyist, as she liked to make out, but because she was an *appearance professional*—she had a knack for picking table runners and nice blouses, but she was also schooled in consumer behavior and the science of desire, innately grasping that beauty does a lot more for human beings than attract sexual partners* or reflect what an individual likes. Aubrey knew what Louis XIV and the Dowager Empress Cixi and Marie Antoinette and Imelda Marcos all knew: that summer palaces and sky-high wigs and twenty-seven hundred pairs of shoes are all stand-ins for power. Beauty is so often power's bitch, particularly in a nonviolent female society like the female expatriate community we all lived in, where husbands footed the bill for competitive domesticity but were usually absent or uninvolved. As I sat on the floor with the unthreatening pile of babies, surrounded by guests agog over Aubrey's interior decor, I realized she was no garden-variety appearance professional, either, but at the top of the heap. She was one of those people who translated her society's unspoken rules into things everyone could see. She was a tastemaker for the tribe.

Part of me felt a little superior, refusing to play the beauty game in the castle of the high priestess. I'd never guessed that skipping the mascara could be so subversive, but it felt the tiniest bit like lying down in front of a tank and singing "Kumbaya." The other part of me, though, felt lonely. I certainly wasn't helping Hattie learn how to share and make nice and turn opponents into friends, just as I wasn't making any professional or social connections for myself. I wasn't

* Good looks have been proven to protect individuals against fear of criticism and suspicion in cases of shoplifting, speeding, and cheating on exams and to lessen reporting and penalization of these crimes. Good looks can also win you arguments, personal confidences, room on the bus, social ease, assertive skill, better grades, shorter waits in line, a feeling of control over your life, and the appearance of intelligence, creativity, marital happiness, mental health, gainful employment, and adventurousness in bed. (On this last point, the assumption is reputedly true—good lookers do get better action.)

even backing John up in his bid to escape an awkward conversation by the chips.

I got up off the floor and milled around. I got a drink and forced a conversation with one of the big-necklace women. As John and I stood at the edge of the gathering, awkwardly knocking elbows and waiting for cake so we could leave, I heard the Voice.

You can't choose not to play this game, she murmured to me. *You can only break the rules and live with the consequences.*

THAT NIGHT, I SAT GLUMLY ON THE JUICE-STAINED COUCH IN MY own Ikea showroom. It was hard to push off the suspicion that a family would be much happier and better adjusted in a home as beautiful as Aubrey's. I might be happier, too, with my old hair and a better wardrobe. Aubrey's attitude toward me was pretty sharp, but she'd never really waved her beauty power in my face; I'd noticed it on my own and had envied it.

This made me think deeply about whether instead of embarking on my experiment I should have just racked up a few thousand dollars in credit-card debt and gone out to purchase my own beauty package: the good-hair headdress, the suit of designer armor, the department-store war paint in shimmering pinks and reds, and the silk throw pillows. Maybe I should have even asked Aubrey to become my personal shopper. At times my inner Voice sure thought this was the way to go. Had I gone in that direction, I might have felt a lot better. I certainly would have looked better. I'd be a bigger hit at tribal gatherings like the birthday party, and I might never have had that terrible moment in the fancy shopwindow.

But in my own way, I'd already tried that route. I'd spent the exorbitant amount on the fancy red dress, and it left me bereft. At the beginning of my experiment, I *knew* I didn't have the resources, time, or cash to be like Aubrey, so I tried her opposite. It had been interesting and informative, but was it so much better?

Six and a half months into my experiment, I knew a lot about what I *didn't* want. I didn't want a static identity that hinged on only one thing, like my hair. I didn't want beauty habits—like slathering on concealer—to obscure real truths about my mental or physical health. I was also tired of living with a mean-girl doppelgänger in the mirror who chronically undermined my best efforts, and I didn't want someone or something else to use my body as a message board. Finally, I wasn't so keen on living in a world where women found their power and worth mainly in their looks and possessions.

What I *did* want was more elusive. There wasn't a clear picture of it out there for me to point at and say, "Yes, that's it!" Although I might have been working toward a more flexible female identity, authentic good health, and a positive self-image not based around the ten minutes in eighth grade when I'd been a buxom size 2—I wasn't there yet. As far as power and worth, frankly, I was really lost. I'd recently pitched a parenting column to a local magazine and had it rejected, and my novel was foundering on some unidentified problem at its core. The liberal arts education I'd spent years amassing meant zero in the context of Important Business-World Transactions. Being a parent gave me power over one tiny person, but this was inconsequential compared to the power Hattie had over me. My income had decreased steadily as I left lower-paying jobs to go along with John to higher-paying ones, and with this move to Hong Kong and Hattie's birth, my financial dependence had become complete.

That night I pulled out my journal. A few weeks earlier, I'd put into words—for the first time—a fantasy of one day owning a closet of beautiful, well-tailored clothes. I dreamed, very concretely, of being a "well-dressed woman," someone others would acknowledge and admire. One of my most coveted items was a leather handbag, something sleek and functional that did not say "discount," or "funky," or "market in Thailand," but "important grown woman," or even "valuable."

As I sat in the quiet apartment that night, I could read the very clear longing for power, relevance, respect, and importance between my words. But this need was incredibly mixed up with a longing for female beauty, even subsumed by it. Looking like a million bucks would be nice, I admitted, but wouldn't earning a million be nicer? Didn't I want professional respect and a meaningful life as much as I wanted a pretty face?

I thought I did. Yet when I envisioned my own empowerment, the best I could come up with was myself wearing a really nice outfit, holding a drop-dead *gorgeous* leather purse.

Snapshot: *The Battle and the Bridge*

New Jersey, Summer and Fall 2010; Boston, October 2011

One of the first things I noticed when we got back to the States was how easy it was to spot a woman whose beauty power had failed. The media led the charge: there was furor over Supreme Court nominee Elena Kagan's haircut (dull? mannish? boring?) that threatened to overwhelm coverage of her views. News of Kate Middleton's weight loss quickly dominated tabloids that had just crowned her a queen of kindness and taste. But it wasn't just the chattering class that remarked on these blunders. When John and I caught the end of a *60 Minutes* piece on Hillary Clinton one night, he said with characteristic bluntness, "Wow, she looks really old." I couldn't scold him because my knee-jerk reaction had been the same, although I held my tongue. Morely Safer, no dewy picture of youth himself, got none of our scrutiny. This same double standard seemed clearest to me in a *New Yorker* photo essay of world leaders gathered at the United Nations. The men, Obama, Ahmadinejad, and many others, were given close-up black-and-white portraits in which every mole, pore, and chin whisker was visible. The female leaders were all given three-quarter-length portraits, their faces in soft focus, and their pastel or colored outfits on display.*

"Okay," admitted John when I pointed this out. "I see what you're saying. But you have to be looking for it; otherwise . . . "

Otherwise, it's a bias that's very hard to notice, even in yourself.

We all know it's there, of course, and did even before Naomi Wolf pointed out the "Professional Beauty Qualification" back

* Only one male leader sported a visibly constructed public image to rival the women: Mu'ammar Gadhafi, in drapey peach beige with matching pancake makeup and drawn-on eyebrows.

in 1991.* Twenty years later, women's global earnings are projected to grow by five trillion dollars in the next five years and for the first time in human history, women are poised to take the world's economic reins at the same rate as men. I had these facts in mind when I designed my survey, trusting it would give me an updated and more optimistic perspective on female beauty power.

When the stats started to roll in, I felt like hapless Neo comprehending the full extent of the Matrix for the first time. Nearly three-quarters of my survey respondents felt bested by another woman's "beauty package" when the competition was not for sex or male attention but for something else entirely. Those with lower household incomes felt this beauty competition more. According to the Bureau of Labor Statistics in the 2009 American Time Use Survey, women spend an extra thirteen minutes per day on their appearance, ostensibly trying to live up to an entrenched belief system shared by men and women alike that female good grooming is necessarily more involved, important, and expensive than men's and usually includes makeup, heels, jewelry, facelifts when appropriate, and colored or highlighted hair.† It would be hard to argue against a woman's right to do this primping—but having the right to do something and *wanting* to do it are different things. When I asked my female survey takers about this, the majority responded that they felt uncomfortable with different standards of grooming for men and women in the public sphere.

* This is the catch-22 that requires a woman to maintain a high level of attractiveness in the workplace but not be so pretty that she causes her male colleagues to drop their manila folders and molest her.

† A great example of this grooming differential was the razzing presidential candidate John Edwards received for a $400 haircut in 2007, while vice presidential candidate Sarah Palin was publicly excused for spending $10,000 for two weeks of hairstyling and $22,800 for a personal makeup artist in the same period.

Survey Questions

How comfortable do you feel about the difference in standards of grooming for men and women in the public sphere?

Very uncomfortable	33%
A little uncomfortable	26%
Conflicted	15%
Mostly comfortable	11%
Very comfortable	10%
Other	6%

Have you ever felt bested by another woman because she had a better "beauty package" even when you were not competing for a sexual partner?

Yes	71%
No	26%
Other	6%

Percentage of respondents in each income bracket who felt bested by another woman's "beauty package":

Less than $50,000	71%
$50,000–100,000	76%
$100,000–500,000	63%
over $500,000	49%

"It's still such a mess!"

This is what I say to a new girlfriend and neighbor of mine one autumn morning in Boston as we are walking home after dropping kids at school. What I'm talking about is an unfinished chapter, but what I really mean is the difficult intersection of female good looks, power, and self-worth. Mandy nods knowingly, no stranger to this material. Just like Aubrey, she's an appearance professional, a stylist about to leave her youngest with a sitter and head off to her clients at an upscale hair salon. This once might have caused tension between us, but by now I've come to realize that I'm an appearance professional, too, because of this book. We're all appearance professionals to some degree or another, trying to look sharp, or capable or sexy or serious, in a bewildering array of venues: at home, at the office, in front of the audience, behind the podium, on the court, in the classroom, on duty, and after hours. Everybody's playing this beauty game, but every one of us has our favorite cheats and laughing about them robs the rules of their power.

"You'll get it," Mandy encourages me as we part ways, and so I head up to my desk this warm fall morning and spread out my various approaches like so many fallen leaves: data, notes, anecdotes, magazine clippings, even a battle scene I wrote last summer in classic Hong Kong kung-fu style: a plain-Jane reactionary (me) takes on the all-powerful Beauty Queen (Aubrey) in hand-to-hand domestic combat. Thinking about the failure of this silly scene—it refused to end, and no one could win because we kept sitting down to swap notes—I do get it, finally. When you pit women against beauty, no one wins. And also: when you pit women against women, it's hard to tell how anyone is doing. The fight ends up less like kung fu than capoeira, that under-the-radar cross between competitive fighting and cooperative dance. All the moves, even the aggressive ones, are still made in a common shadow—in this case, a not-so-distant female past. Many of us—myself included—are still standing in a spot between being valued and being taken for granted, between independence and connection, between domestic concern and worldly participation, and between acting powerfully and feeling loved. Whether we cultivate or reject it, the beauty package is one of many steps across a bridge between the old world of womanhood and the new.

If the first half of my experiment showed me this bridge I was crossing, then the second half of my experiment posed a new and more difficult challenge. How was I supposed to stand on a narrow plank amid all this movement, change, and turmoil—with the sky above, the water below, my child pulling on my hand, history and family calling to me from behind, my friends racing on ahead—and be happy?

How was I to find beauty in a tumultuous passage, and in the person making it?

8

Pretty Mind

For a lack of attention a thousand forms of loveliness elude us every day.

—Evelyn Underhill, early-twentieth-century Christian mystic and writer

Hong Kong, September and October 2007

A half mile behind the Bon Point building lay the Morning Path. This east-facing trail snaked uphill through Lung Fu Shan country park toward Victoria Peak, and although it was wide, paved, and usually filled with joggers and dog walkers, it still felt wild to me as it twisted through a dripping and verdant jungle.* During our stay in Hong Kong, I walked it as often as I could.

As the weather cooled to tolerable fall temperatures, and as my experiment moved into its second half, I sometimes walked as often as twice a week. I would begin on a fitness

* It *was* a little wild. The *South China Morning Post* occasionally featured articles on how to free errant pets from the coils of Burmese pythons.

mission—sometimes with Hattie, sometimes without—but always accompanied by the Voice's carping: *You should get an odometer to track your progress. You should get a heart-rate monitor.* It wasn't just my heart rate that bothered her, though. She was also hurt, angry, and confused about what was happening. *Look, you're just a good person who's been sidetracked by appearances, not some woman struggling with your own ambition, competitiveness, or tendencies to judge! No one has any power, you know. That's why therapy and mind-altering substances were invented! And if beauty is so relative and out of your control, why not just go along with whatever it is wherever you are? You can learn to love shaggy haircuts and bubble dresses. You know, you said things would be better by now, and they've only gotten more confusing.*

I listened to this monologue as I pumped uphill, but didn't have any answers.

Luckily, by the time I passed the turnoff for the old World War II arsenal, the Voice had usually become winded, like me—and I could pause to look down over the steep hillside and across the tips of skyscrapers, or watch one of Hong Kong's 235 species of butterfly: the Indian Cabbage White or the Great Eggfly with royal blue at the tips of black wings. The Morning Path ended at Lugard Road, an elevated stone thoroughfare that ringed the Peak. My favorite section was a long stretch of earthbound road that hugged the mountainside, concealing gates to precarious mansions and shaded by massive banyan trees.

I knew I was not the first to be inspired by the banyans' giant rooty tendrils, or ability to weather-signal eight typhoons,* but as

* The Hindu god Krishna reputedly sat in one while he created the universe, and Buddha attained enlightenment under a banyan. Despite its nasty nickname (strangler fig) and bad reputation as an invasive species, the banyan is printed on the Indonesian coat of arms, believed to bestow good fortune at Hong Kong's own Lam Tsuen wishing trees, and generally revered across Asia.

I gazed up into the gnarled branches and reddish leaves one morning, I thought I might have been the first to be *jealous* of them. I envied most their lack of consciousness. They simply reacted to whatever arose: a drought, a crowded hillside, or an invasive beetle. They had no troublesome feelings about these issues. They were just living, while I was mired in *thinking* about living.

My stated intent for my treks up the Morning Path was to shape up my cardiovascular system and my rear end. What they really did was shape up my brain. They gave me a break from all the conflicting things it said. They called my attention to the stories I always told myself that just weren't coming true.

THE FIRST OF THESE STORIES, I FELT, WAS THE ONE ABOUT HOW TWO financially stable, consenting adult partners and a healthy baby should look and act like a happy family. John had recently been commended at work, an accomplishment I secretly dreaded because it only drove him to work harder and longer to prove that he was worth the praise. His work travel had taken a sharp uptick that fall. I had plenty of mom-and-baby company during daylight, but nighttime in our apartment became a nadir of aloneness. Dinner was especially nasty, as I insisted on a shared meal of hard-to-prepare health foods, and Hattie reacted with furiously hungry wailing, culinary skepticism, and sometimes gleeful spit-outs.*

After these terrible dinners, Hattie and I would leave the wreckage on the table and take our mango or lychee or Hami

* I'm definitely not the first to harp on this domestic valley of shadow: for the suicidal version, see "Lesbos" in Sylvia Plath's *Ariel*.

melon out to our balcony, where I'd laid a cotton mat on the ground. (No chairs for us; there were stories of children using them to climb over rails and then shinny down drainpipes, and I didn't want Hattie getting any ideas.) We'd peer through the balcony railing at the harbor as the pungent scents of more appealing dinners in other apartments wafted by. These desserts were nice, but I'd expected "having a family" to look like some Norman Rockwell–ish Sunday supper, with a pile of biscuits on the table and the beloved pup catching scraps beneath everyone's feet. Hattie loved watching the red-sailed tourist sampan cruise into the sunset; I watched the same thing with empty melancholy.

But life is good! That was the second story I was wrestling with. I knew I *should* have felt that way, but sometime between Hattie's birth and now, my life had turned into a Sisyphean to-do list. Trips to the beach were ruined by the equipment management they required and the schedule they upset; my work demanded concentration I didn't have and skills I couldn't find time to get. Even if I saw that my life had compressed itself into a Möbius loop of difficulty and frustration, that gave me no insight whatsoever into what to do about it.

This loop became drastically worse the week John's parents came to visit from Los Angeles. We all went sightseeing in Yangshuo, a scenic destination in the Li River Valley in Mainland China. It was a short, easy trip to a touristy location, a trip I once would have been thrilled to take. Instead, I went safety berserk. I freaked out over the death-trap crib provided by the hotel. When we rented bikes, I balked at the harnessless Easter basket Hattie was supposed to ride in (*unhelmeted?*) as we wove through busy streets. I blanched at the utter lack of seat belts in any vehicle (*Why did we even bring the car seat? We're all going to die anyway*) and stood rigid with my eyes closed as we were shoved with a thronging mob of tourists through a narrow entrance into an unlit cave (*Just push me and my baby into the void, and bury us already*). Worst of all, I could tell that John was siding with his parents the whole time. He believed Mainland China was not actively trying to kill us.

It wasn't until I called a friend in the States and did a blow-by-blow postmortem on this trip that my mood began to take a recognizable shape.

"Are you getting regular periods yet?" Kelly asked with the directness and intuition of a friend of twenty years. "Your voice has an edge I haven't ever heard before."

I'd just had my first postpartum period, during the trip. It had been painful, extremely heavy, and long. I'd come prepared, but bathrooms were few and far between, often squatters or latrines, and dependably filled with flies. Every woman knows that travel and menstruation don't go so well together, but this was menstruation like I'd never known it and travel in a region that made the realities of female hygiene in the developing world shockingly clear. As Kelly and I delved further, I realized it wasn't just this one cycle that had made me crazy but the whole transition from pregnancy to lactation and then back to fertility, as one set of hormones withdrew and another surged into action. This process had taken months, and neither my male OB or female GP had breathed a word of the psychological toll it might take or how when combined with chronic fatigue and new-parenting stress, these hormones might turn to killer bees in my bonnet, wrecking the normal movement of my mind.

Fortunately, Kelly—who worked in television, not medicine—had a sensible prescription for me. I promised to read up on postpartum depression and premenstrual dysphoric disorder and call her back if I thought my symptoms matched up. (They didn't.) I was to consider cutting Hattie off from breast-feeding right away and start the Pill, although I was sure my opinionated female GP would dissuade me. At my last visit she'd instructed, "You must conceive your second child as soon as the first is weaned. Difficult for you, but this is the best way for them." This clarified for me, in case I'd missed it, that my own concerns were purely secondary.

A final option was to put Hattie in a helmet, shin guards, and a flak jacket and lock all the apartment doors and windows until I'd arranged to move back from Hong Kong. "I'll get right on that," I told Kelly, and we both laughed, although really I just felt the relief of comprehension.

MY AUNT, A COMMITTED PRACTITIONER OF ZEN BUDDHISM, SENT ME a book that fall. It was a parenting book by a woman who had been a member of a Zen monastery and then become a first-time parent in her forties. I didn't feel I had much use for this personal growth/self-help book, yet I read it the way one drinks blue Gatorade after thirty-six hours of food poisoning—my cherished personal objections becoming irrelevant in the deliciousness of its functionality. As I read the book, I was reminded that in graduate school, I'd relied on a semiregular meditation practice to dull the sting of days when I understood myself to be an admissions mistake. And so one night I got out a candle and the brass singing bowl I picked up in Vietnam. I sat cross-legged in our bedroom window seat with my back straight, a pillow tucked under my butt, my eyes unfocused at a vague spot six inches away from my knees, and my hands in the meditation mudra, the shape of infinity and openness.

After forty-five seconds, my jaw went slack, and I fell asleep. I jerked myself awake, assumed my position with much more resolve, and promptly fell asleep again. I blew out the candle, got into bed, and stayed up late reading—sullenly—about how much meditation can help people at wit's end.

The next night I caffeinated myself. I didn't nod off and did manage to count my breaths past six, but instead of calm, I got more chatter about my problems, courtesy of the Voice.

I can't believe your OB didn't give you a postpartum-depression screen. Hello! This is not the fifties!

Innnnnnn and Ouuuut. Breath one and breath two.

I mean, you got some of the best medical care available in Asia! What about all those women having babies over on the Mainland or in Vietnam? What do you think is going unnoticed or unchecked or crappily stitched up in them?

I pretended not to be interested.

You fucking should be interested! Why is it that you think of motherhood as a path to personal fulfillment instead of a basic human chore? Who told you labor and childbirth were an opportunity for self-expression? And if you're looking for inner peace and happiness, then why are you being such a hard-assed drill sergeant about everything? You want to be self-disciplined about your work, self-disciplined about health and exercise, self-disciplined about not using plastic bags and buying organic—and now, on top of it all, you have to be disciplined about beauty? You've given up pretty hair so you can obsess about a pretty MIND?

Yes.

Come on! It's really hard to be woman, and it's really hard to be you!

I didn't listen to whiners. These thoughts were simply clouds passing through my mind.

They ain't passing, sister. I got a six-month supply of unused estrogen right here telling me to sit tight.

I gave up on the meditation. Whatever she was fueled by right now, the Voice of complaint was just too loud to contend with or wait out. And while she was annoying, accusatory, and defensive all at once, I felt she had valid points, maybe even all valid points. Harping on them, however, solved nothing and gave me no peace.

"Your life is a garden," the Zen parenting book said. "And you are the only gardener." Maybe this was so, but during the year of my experiment, I just couldn't see it that way. I felt the garden was elsewhere, out on the Morning Path, hidden deep inside the vegetative awareness of the banyan trees, or located somewhere in the future when all the problems of all the world's women (starting with my own) were solved. I insisted—and the Voice in my head backed me up 100 percent—that my problems lay with John's job, my weakness for skin-care products, the expatriate lifestyle, an archaic medical establishment ignorant of female experience, a sensitive and sleepless kid, and the last hundred pages of my novel. And the solution to all these problems was the story I told myself about beauty—both inner and outer. I believed it was something out there, and attainable, if only I could improve myself enough to gain its blessing. I was very attached to this beauty story because I thought it was all I had.

Snapshot: *Trees and Ponds*

Concord, Massachusetts, 2011

On a brilliant, cool morning in late October, John and I drive the kids out to Concord for a walk around Walden Pond. On the banks of this pond, Henry David Thoreau threw off the bonds of civilization and took to the woods "to live deliberately . . . and not, when [he] came to die, discover that [he] had not lived." I'm excited to see the small, self-made cabin, even if it's only a reproduction, but when we arrive, the adjacent parking lot is jammed with cars. I fret, but John stays cool and we find a spot. We head around the pond on a woodsy, unpaved path, and as the stroller hits gnarled roots, I wince. Five years and two kids have turned my scorn for "overcivilized" hiking into appreciation for sidewalks.

We make slow, bumpy progress, stopping occasionally to throw stones in. Fringed by scarlet leaves, the bright, still pond looks beautiful to me. But I'm also aware that today, each of us is projecting our own story upon its emerald surface: the story of easy parking and literary sightseeing (me), the story of an athletic warm-up to hearty fall lunch (John), and the story of innocence and an unjust reprimand (Hattie, who gets yelled at after nearly pushing John in). Orson, at two and a half, is the only one of us who meets Walden Pond where it lives: in its wetness and splashiness. Halfway around, even he comes up with a pond story that has to be curtailed—the story of a wild forest boy swinging a pointed stick near people's eyes. Our stories delight us intensely, yet often fail us, or come to an end.

I saw straight through my own beauty story very briefly, in the fall of 2010. Orson was already a year and a half old. Like anyone going up to bat a second time, I'd invented some inspiring motivational tales about how things would go in my second child's babyhood: better sleep habits, better mealtimes, better attitude, better everything. Eighteen months in, my inner sales pitches were failing me, and the chaos was still expanding like a mushroom cloud. From experience I knew meditation was beyond me as a sleep-deprived baby mama, so I turned to a book of Zen koans instead.

The idea of a koan is that you run a piece of verbal nonsense through your head until sense and nonsense trade places and offer up insight. For all of us who like to butt our heads against something, the answerless riddle of a koan is an ideal wall. The bonus is that no staying awake on a soft cushion in a quiet room is required. You can work on a koan while pushing a swing or washing a dish. The koan I began with was this:

Does a dog have Buddha nature?

No.

I started repeating this Q&A in my mind while I diapered, folded laundry, and shopped for chicken breast. After a week or so of unproductive repetition, I started thinking that "Buddha nature" was pretty much equivalent to "inner beauty," and so I subbed in those words, instead.

Does a dog have inner beauty?

No.

Is a dog beautiful?

No.

I was dismayed by how negative this riddle solving was, and how cruel. Why was "No" kicking the poor dog? Frustrated by my lack of progress, I tried switching the subject around, too, so that I became the dog.

When I try to stay patient with the kids, is that inner beauty?

No.

When I buy used snow pants to economize is that Buddha nature?

No.

Sometimes I couldn't believe how hard "No" was riding my ass. How could it be that even with my very best efforts at being an attentive mom and wife—at staying in the game professionally, at vanquishing the yard work and paperwork, at sending the relatives pictures of the kids in a timely fashion, and not freaking out at my husband when he couldn't figure out where he was going to move us to next—the answer was still **No?** My writing? **No.** My education? **No.** My hopes, even for health and love and peace in the world? **No. No. No. Not beautiful. Not Buddha nature.** I decided that koans were for masochists and people with better senses of self-worth than I. I told **No** to go to hell, but it kept running through my mind like a spiritually nasty pop song, endlessly repeating its downer mantra.

My fight with **No** ended one cold fall morning as I took Orson for a walk to Kelley Pond. This small, man-made runoff basin was hidden in the woods behind a nearby elementary school. It was a convenient nature walk, if imperfect: I didn't like to pass the muddy town mulch area to get there, and the woods were not thick enough to hide the plastic toys in people's backyards. That day, though, the water in the pond was bright and clear, and the surrounding trees were decked out in autumnal finery. I looked at the long grass tilting at the bank, still a summer green. Orson stared quietly at the yellow, red, and brown trees and mirrorlike water, rapt.

Is this pond beautiful?

Does it have Buddha nature?

No.

If this pond isn't beautiful, my brain screamed at the koan, *then nothing is!*

With that, the word *beauty* dissolved. It cleared to the edges of my understanding like grease moving away from a drop of soap. And in the clean, empty center that remained were just the plain things themselves: the water in the pond, the deleafing trees, the breeze carrying vapors of pine and compost, the bright dots of sun on the toes of Orson's boots. I looked from the pond to a pile of discarded beer cans in the undergrowth and found I had no feelings of comparison or preference for either one. I didn't wish the traffic noise away; it was okay with me. I looked down at my hands, too—dry, cold, and veined, resting on the stroller's handles. The knuckles were raw, and palest pink. The realness of my hands surprised me, as did the pulse I could feel inside.

That moment of realization was a powerful shock—my brain would always draw me to what it knew as beautiful and would always give those things special value, but that brain itself was acculturated, hormonal, self-referential, and hardwired in certain limiting ways. It was deeply marvelous to draw my own mental software aside like a curtain—even for an instant—and peek at a whole universe unbound by my classifications, judgments, language, or beloved stories.

We do live in a world filled with these stories: success stories, love stories, stories of redemption and failure. The good ones can help us grow, or point us in the right direction. In the years since my experiment, I've worked on creating a new story of beauty for myself—one inspired by the rings of a banyan tree, with the gift of life at the core, and the delight of art and artifice at the outermost edge. But even a good story can set us up to hold reality at gunpoint, waiting for the promised payoff: *I need youth or a semblance of it!* the Voice rails. *I need happiness or self-worth or inner peace! I need my life to be better than it is, and I will do whatever it takes to make it that way—just give me the ten-step program!* But just as caffeine doesn't solve a chronic sleep debt, stories of ambitious self-improvement don't address the reality of a chaotic and imperfect world. Sometimes the gardens of our lives become stroller-unfriendly jungles filled with pet-snatching Burmese pythons. And what then? Raze the forest and unroll the Astroturf?

The more effective approach, I'm beginning to see, is to embrace the paradise that is already here: my real, living body; my real children; and my real husband. All of us are more deserving of my best effort than the phantoms of perfection: the children I hope I am raising, the husband I sometimes wish I had, the woman I feel I should be.

Survey Question

Which of the following do you rely on most often to bring more beauty into your life?

Loved ones or humanity in general	71%
The natural physical world	65%
The arts	44%
Home and things I own	37%
The universal or divine	18%
Work and the problems I solve	17%
Other	4%

A Language Every Body Speaks

Remember that always dressing in understated good taste is the same as playing dead.

—SUSAN CATHERINE, ACTRESS

HONG KONG, NOVEMBER 2007

In November, my experiment hit a plateau. I'd had bad hair for so long that a "bad-hair day" meant nothing to me. My face without makeup now said "face" to me, not "hideous problem," and I'd outed chronic fatigue, professional confusion, and raging hormones. Still, I was restless. I wanted to shake things up on the appearance front in the last months. My experiment had yielded some big surprises, but I wanted to go deeper still, confronting any rules that seemed beyond questioning.

My clothes, for example, and the way I wore them. My clothes had triggered all my worst insecurities in the months before my experiment, but as I sat on the end of the bed looking at them one fall morning, I realized my approach to getting dressed hadn't changed a bit. I hadn't purchased anything new (save the swimsuit and—full disclosure—one two-dollar hot-pink tank top), but I still labored mightily to produce the same averagely appropriate conformist outfits. And although I didn't get stuck in the mirror as often, getting dressed was still a cross between playing chess and saying "I love you"—an endeavor both intimate and strategic that never felt like a full success to me and almost always triggered nasty commentary from the Voice. Yes, everyone wore clothes, and yes, everyone thought about them a little bit, but my clothes seduced, punished, comforted, and betrayed me. If it was power I was looking for, my clothes had it . . . over me. Here, I thought, was a nice, messy Pandora's box to dump out.

By now I knew I could look bad and live on—and even enjoy it a little. I'd partied in one of Hong Kong's trendiest bars plainface, I'd worn a bra top to a wedding, I'd kept my cool without any beauty armor at all in front of Aubrey the mean girl, and I'd not yet lost a friend to my unstyled mushroom head. Flush with these small but personally significant victories, I decided to set myself free of fashion constraints—at least my own and those on the streets of Hong Kong. After all, my outfits rarely delighted me, and I wasn't so down with Hong Kong's more-is-more aesthetic: a typical women's T-shirt was embellished with at least two of the following: ribbons, pearls, bells, leatherette embossed leaves, silk embroidery, jewels, zippers, and feathers on long strings.

I'd deliberately quit shopping for my experiment, but I'd never considered not getting myself dressed at all. Not going nude, just . . . not choosing. Maybe John could pick my outfits for the day! I'd always marveled at his ability to clothe himself without ever doubting his choice or changing his mind. I might end up wearing the soft, shapeless knit comfortwear that John dressed Hattie in and wore himself during every hour he did not have to wear a suit, but so what?

But it was not so easy for me to ask John for a favor, even this small one. The awkward trip to the Li River with his parents had raised a host of long-winded, possibly accusatory, talking points between us: family loyalty, fear, the way parenthood seemed to have sapped my general trust in the world. A brief pregnancy scare shortly thereafter had terrified John and made me question whether I wanted to bring another child into an already overstretched family living in an overcrowded world that lacked seat belts. We needed to talk through all of this, but John had projects in China, Singapore, and Korea that fall and a conference in Barcelona. Between butt-numbing flights, he stumbled home but then had to decompress for twelve hours at least, first as a set of glazed-over eyes in front of the tube, then as a plasma blob under the bedclothes. When he awoke from these recovery periods, he reached for me under the covers, snuggled with Hattie, and told us about the far-away city where he'd been. Then the alarm would go off for the second or third time, and he would become an automaton sweeping aside bedclothes and marching himself into the shower. The twelve minutes of John's getting dressed on a workday morning: this was what we had, and there was no room inside it for grievances, let alone daily favors.

One of these mornings I did mention my experiment's plateau to the cloud of steam escaping from the bathroom. "So, to push this envelope, I'm thinking of paring down my wardrobe to only two or three outfits," I said. "I think the trick might be to eliminate the hell of choice. I'll be like you. I'll wear the same exact thing every day."

"You're turning into a monk," said the cloud. "Maybe you should write a comedy about a stay-at-home dad who is also a monk."

"Why not a stay-at-home mom?" I joked. "Can't women be as funny as men?"

He didn't say anything. I knew he was getting tired of my experiment's game. If, after eight months, this experiment wasn't making me inwardly satisfied and outwardly radiant, then what the hell was the point? He'd found the idea of becoming a plain Jane interesting, but he didn't really understand all these "women's issues" I was yammering about suddenly, as if *I* had the hard job sitting around in a nice apartment all day and he was a big jerk.

I didn't think he was a jerk. If I did, I wouldn't have missed him so much.

"I'm not turning into a monk," I said quietly. "More like Emily Dickinson." I chuckled to myself, having a private joke about my total lack of poetic ability—although the poetess and I did share a fondness for white clothing. And surely the simple, white housedress she wore daily for twenty years had been a neat trick—the clothing equivalent of a Zen koan. By eliminating variation and choices in one realm, she had freed herself to more effectively confront another: sartorial stooge becomes grammatical genius. Dickinson's ankle-length long-sleeved dress was hardly the all-in-one for playground outings in the tropics, though. A much better uniform might be the loose, floral poly-blend pajama ensemble worn by tiny, antique Cantonese ladies all over Hong Kong—never mind the fact that it would make me look eighty-five. While the uniform seemed a good long-term solution to the problem of clothing choice, it did require some up-front investment and research—neither of which I wanted to make.

John was not a monk, either, but he got dressed just as easily as one—without hesitation or indecision. When he emerged from his cloud of steam, he applied his pin-striped uniform with automatic motions. He tied his tie without the help of a mirror, drew on his dark socks, levered his feet into his shoes, and was out the door without breakfast, coffee, or a newspaper, leaving on my cheek something less like a kiss than a distracted promise that one day—when he'd made partner maybe, or when he felt financially secure, or maybe not even until he retired—we'd get around to our lives, and to each other.

Although I couldn't have articulated it to either of us just then, the questions my experiment was posing seemed to expose how keenly our worlds were opposed: John's workaday world seemed to depend on an absence of personhood and personal life, a requirement that was reflected in his hours, his travel, and even in his standard-issue suits. In contrast, my new world of domesticity seemed to be powered by a magnification of personhood and personal life: a couch could never just be a couch, and an outfit could never just be clothes; these things were actually *me*. John's predicament made me sad for our family and for families everywhere. My own predicament made me angry. Why couldn't pants just be pants? Why couldn't a shirt just keep off the sun?

I could do better, I thought. Skipping makeup, jewelry, hairdos, and shopping options had gained me hundreds of minutes a year. How much more might I gain without fashion to worry about? And if I could go there, might I also get to a whole life untroubled by the problem of pleasing aesthetics—a world in which sheets remained unmatched, gardens were filled with blooming weeds, and dish towels went from a wad in the dryer to a wad in the drawer without being neatly folded up on the way? I shuddered to think of this grim practical universe, but hungering for beauty in every corner of life was a chronic time and money suck. Sure, my day could be sent in the right direction by the sun on a decorative handblown glass vase, but I wanted to be able to ignore that vase when I had to.

So. If I wasn't going to wear a uniform, and I wasn't going to let John pick, I *could* simply put clothes on myself the way I took bus fare out of the pewter bowl near our door: randomly. That morning, I tried it. I stood before my wardrobe and closed my eyes, letting my fingers wander across the shoulders of my blouses. From the heft of the fabric I figured I could choose a weather-appropriate outfit. I pinched the shoulder of something cotton and bumpy. My turquoise eyelet shirt.

Nope, too hard to coordinate with. Try the sundress.

I deliberately searched for the rough, light drape of one of my favorites, but once I'd done that, the game was up. I couldn't do randomness; my fingers already knew too much.*

Instead, I settled for deliberate badness: let me pair this hot-pink plaid skirt with this blue-and-red tank top and see

* Chances are John wouldn't have had the same problem with his clothes; studies have recently found a higher density of nerve endings in women's fingers than in men's.

what happens. To my amazement, when I stood ready to go and waiting in the mirrored elevator lobby, I got a nod of approval from a reflection I barely recognized. I stared at an art-student hipster who knew the name of every underground dance club in Kowloon, owned several pairs of hand-crocheted leg warmers, and gagged at the thought of monogrammed bathrobes.

You just shaved off five years, said the Voice approvingly.

Interesting. Just as the habit of concealing my fatigue with undereye makeup could cover up my potential for true restedness and health, perhaps my assumptions about "correct" outfits could mask the expressive potential of my clothes. I may not have been up to Central Hong Kong's dressy standards, but I did go off to my appointment with a cooler-than-thou swagger.

The next day, it didn't go as well. In preparation for a playdate, I dressed myself in an olive-green shirt and a pair of pants in a browner shade. I wore sneakers; I left the shirt untucked. I felt uncertain as we left the building and fretful in the cab. Later, Corinne asked me, "Are you sure you're feeling all right today? You look a bit gray."

"Off day," I replied bleakly, and as the hours passed, it became one. I felt worse and worse. When Hattie and I got home and spotted ourselves in our own mirrored elevator lobby, Hattie's bright-purple romper prompted her to smile. I squinted at myself with a bleary clinical eye, wondering whether this woman-zombie before me needed a blood transfusion, some sun, or an antidepressant.

Okay, fine. I could do inappropriate (armpit hair, nasty old sandals), and I could do ugly (mushroom head), but I just couldn't do olive bland—not without something else, like a bright scarf—to counteract it. I'd known that color psychology was a big part of marketing and packaging design (fast food wrapped in appetite-enhancing red and orange; ecofriendly detergents bottled in morally pristine white), but I'd not realized how much it affected me and everyone I encountered. Did I want to feel like Nauseous Kermit and present myself thus? Or did I want to present something, anything, sunnier? This question fatally weakened my resolve to dress badly, and after only three days, I gave up.* It upset me a little that, even this far into the experiment, I was still unwilling to push far past my own boundaries as well as everyone else's. But thinking about this made me wonder if I really knew where any of these boundaries were.

When I examined my closet again, I saw something less like a cohesive wardrobe than a child's overstuffed costume trunk, filled with identities and poses I had tried on, used, and discarded. There were garments for trying to look older and more mature (a peach postcollege interview suit) and for trying to look younger and hipper (blouses from Forever 21). There were designer clothes that fit me poorly but were made well (Italian tweed vest) and thrift-store junk in a bad color that I wore daily because it fit me perfectly and was really useful (navy-blue poly-blend raincoat with snaps and empire seaming). There was an embarrassingly big pile of clothes that said "Hey, boys, I'm available" that were either uncomfortable, impractical, or both.

---

* There have been several fashion experimenters far more successful than I: in 1991 Andrea Zittel designed and wore a series of black-and-white uniforms for six months each in "A–Z Uniforms," in 2005 Alex Martin stitched her own garment for the yearlong "Little Brown Dress Project," and in 2009 Sheena Matheiken raised money for a charity by wearing the same black dress for a year in the "Uniform Project." No male performance artists have done uniform projects to my knowledge, presumably because the public reaction would be "So what?"

Survey Questions

How many items of clothing (including shoes, hats, and underwear) do you acquire in a year?

0–3	2%
3–10	17%
10–20	37%
20–50	33%
50–100	9%
100–200	1%
More than 200	0.6%

Did you play dress up as a child?

Yes	80%
No	20%

Since my effort to dress badly had failed, I went back to a modified Plan A, paring my wardrobe down. I culled old office clothes, bagged-out pregnancy garments, unhappy pleather purses, and things I had to admit I'd never be able to wear again. (Good-bye pale-blue silk sheath with no give, good-bye sweet C-cup brassieres!) As I stacked things up in garbage bags and readied them for the donation bin, I found there were useful things I wanted to scrap as well as utterly frivolous things I hated to abandon. One example was a shiny golden scarf I'd appropriated from a cooler roommate years ago. At eighteen I'd folded that scarf up, pinned it in place, and called it a skirt. At twenty-five I'd worn it as a shawl. Out of a sense of maternal modesty, I'd recently used the scarf as a holiday table runner, not a garment.

Hattie was sitting on the bed near me when I found this scarf, doing elasticity studies with the awful nude pantyhose I'd worn to the Red-Hot party.

"Shred 'em, baby, shred 'em," I told her.

I envied the years of dress-up play still in front of her, and felt sad, too, knowing that someday—maybe around the age of three or four—her delight in clothes would become attention to decorum. She'd be taught, by me probably, that the world's rules about clothing were more important than her own taste. I opened the scarf and flicked it over her toes, made it dance just out of her reach, and tossed it high. As it opened over us like a golden parachute, the two of us lay back on the bed and waited for it to gild us, one delectable inch of skin at a time.

Don't give it away, the Voice said with surprising gentleness. *Some of your selves you can do without, but not this one.*

Was it selves I had stripped from my hangers and dumped into those black plastic garbage bags, or was it only clothes? Whatever lay inside, there were five bags full of it, representing at least twelve or fifteen years and almost as many identities. I could have taken my bags all down to the drop box in King George Park that very day, but I didn't. Instead, I let them sit there, lined up against the wall, waiting.

❧

WHEREAS I OWNED AND USED CLOTHES, "FASHION" WAS SOMETHING else, a force that repelled me as much as it beguiled. Throughout my experiment, I watched the television show *Project Runway.* This habit was ideologically inconvenient and contrary to all the principles I was pledged to uphold, yet I flicked it on weekly and watched it from the doorway of the kitchen, supposedly doing something else. I argued to myself that in watching clothing designers work up a garment, I was watching art being shaped (and routinely smashed) by market forces. From that point of view, I found it dramatic when inspiration trumped skillful technique or when trend trumped what I called beauty—as happened one night when a contestant produced a shirt-and-skirt combo that looked like a bagel falling out of a blue sandwich bag.

"Eww, *look* at that thing!" I cried aloud, and then the brown pouf skirt and unstructured teal blouse garnered raves from every judge. Instances like these reminded me that I knew absolutely zip about what fashion was, what it did, or how it worked. And it was not for lack of paying attention, either.

In my late twenties I'd become a devotee of the magazine "must-have" lists—the ones that admonish us all to have trim pencil skirts, neutral cardies, and ballet flats.* Admittedly, I was a latecomer, but once I found them, I became a habitual checker and cross-checker. Mom came to visit me once, during my period of list infatuation, and when we chatted about the must-haves, she was intrigued. These clothing rules were news to her as well.

Her own mother, a woman we called Sugar, had run away from a farm-girl past in Tacoma, married southern "breeding," and moved to a wealthy suburb on the Eastern Seaboard. Sugar could pull a coat off the rack in a fancy department store, look carefully at it, and then reproduce it on her own sewing machine so skillfully that each of her four daughters could

* I give you an amalgamated version of the Must-Have List: little black dress, crisp white shirt, lightweight cashmere cardigan, perfect dark jeans, classic pumps, trench coat, pencil skirt, all-occasion bag, selection of good T-shirts, ballet flats, fitted blazer, fancy scarf, good suit, black slacks, knee-high boots, statement necklace, lace bra, "dress" pajamas, and khaki pants.

wear it in turn. Sometimes she'd sew a fake label in, just in case. If the message Sugar wanted her girls to send with their clothes was a little anxious, it was very clear: "I am a good girl from a reputable and wealthy family," the clothes said. "Go ahead and check my tag."

The message the must-have list items sent, Mom and I agreed, was totally different. It went something like: "I am young, I have an office job and access to contraception, and I do not ever run, squat, or do anything in foul weather for more than five minutes." Some of the list items might be useful here or there, but on the whole, they were remarkably impractical for a landscape painter, like Mom, or someone who worked on school playgrounds and owned a white dog, like me. At the top of both of our must-have lists? Wide-brimmed sun hats.

But it wasn't the practicality or impracticality of the lists that was important to me back in my twenties. What I loved about them was the suggestion of fail-safe rules in a previously chaotic fashion universe—edicts that I'd never been parentally ingrained with, like "please" and "thank you." Mom and I had a few tussles in my childhood about dresses and tights; she was trying to teach me the good-girl thing but eventually realized it was useless in a small Arizona town where the ministers, bank tellers, and even my teachers at school wore skin-tight Wrangler jeans. As a theatrical teen, I wore oversize military jackets, too-tight skirts, and couch-worthy prints with a smile on my face. When I finally encountered the must-have lists, I was nearing thirty, but they appeared like a set of alphabet blocks to the almost-literate child—promising entry to an urbane adult world.

It was not long after the bagel-and-sandwich bag episode of *Project Runway* that I set out—once and for all—to make sense of fashion's rules, at least on paper. If clothes really did "speak," as people on that show sometimes said they did, then maybe I could decode the "language" of fashion. I sat down on our bed armed with my journal, a few colored pens, and the dregs of what I remembered from a college course in linguistics. (I'd argued to my parents that it would have some practical application besides fulfilling a math requirement, and here it was!) As I boxed out a rough chart, I conjured images of my dad in his Volunteer Fire Department gear, my mom in the floor-length gown she'd had made for our wedding, John in his sharp suits, and me in various fashion disasters. I scribbled and I jotted. I moved things around and crossed out.

Nerdy though it was, my chart was a revelation to me. Fashion really did function just like English, Chinese, French, or Spanish: it had content (words or garments), rules of grammar (how to functionally arrange that content), and room for emotional nuance and personal expression. It was different in different countries but was used to do some of the same things in each and was learned by children right alongside their native tongues.* I felt like the Noam Chomsky of fashion! I began to see how people used clothes to communicate, sometimes weighting one column over another, but ultimately juggling all three.

---

* Interestingly, the very deepest structure of modern clothing's language is sex differentiation. Babies get garments aggressively asserting femininity and masculinity before they can focus their eyes, and by the age of four a girl understands she can choose any garment she likes so long as it adheres to a wide feminine color palette, while a boy is allowed only pants, shorts, and unadorned tops in a strict masculine color palette. The strictness of these rules seems "natural" to us, but it rivals some of the most draconian sartorial codes in history. When the United States was founded, boys wore dresses and hair ribbons until they were six.

The Language of Clothes

1	2	3
What Clothes Do for the Body	**What Clothes Do for a Society**	**What Clothes Do for a Personality**
adjust body temperature repel water repel sun protect skin or organs increase traction or speed carry equipment or kids provide camouflage	cover genitalia cover other body parts for modesty show conformity to norms of grooming and hygiene identify tribal members identify outsiders identify status: age, wealth, profession, education, class, ethnicity threaten aggressor invite sexual advance	reflect mood decorate features broadcast taste, agendas advertise rebellion identify cliques, subgroups, special belonging
And They Do It with . . .	**And They Do It with . . .**	**And They Do It with . . .**
garment features fabric thickness material and fabric engineering	garment type (pants, skirt) garment style (formal, casual) garment cut (relaxed, tailored)	garment color, texture garment body feel garment decoration, pattern, printing, logos garment fit or cleanliness

It wasn't always successfully done, either. Most of us were making grammatical errors all the time. John nailed the social grammar in Column 2 on the weekdays when he wore his perfectly tailored dark suits, but he was often caught in bad weather without a raincoat or umbrella, the right practical gear from Column 1. John also became a fashion "don't" on the weekends, when he OD'd on Column 1. I wished he would occasionally use his clothes to say "Come over here and kiss me" or "This is a great band."

At the bottom of my chart, I wrote: *The Off-Hours Effect = Too Much Column 1.*

Opposite John, on the other far extreme, was Hattie, particularly in her neon-green swimsuit with sharks all over it. It was a flamboyantly expressive Column 3 choice. When I'd looked it over in the shop, I'd worried and had a long moment of doubt as the Voice reinforced some grammatical rules: *Hey! You should dress a female baby like a little girl, not a genderless miniature superhero!* But Hattie's expectant eyes triumphed, and I bought her the suit. All summer, if I hummed the theme from *Jaws,* she'd run to get it. In the elevator lobby on our way down to the pool, she'd grin at herself and stroke her silky arms and belly. "You are amazing," I think the swimsuit said to her, or maybe just "You *are.*" Fashion victimhood was awfully cute in toddlers, but it could look freaky on adults: hemp advocates, high-fashion extremists, medieval recreationists, people who wore Strawberry Shortcake outfits to the dentist.

I wrote: *Too Much Column 3 = "The Magpie Effect"* (named after the bird who lines its nest with shiny trinkets and colorful bits of string).

Both these fashion faux pas stemmed from not paying enough attention to Column 2. Once, early on in our relationship, John had jokingly suggested I avert all Column-2-type fashion disasters by adopting a 100 percent single-retailer wardrobe: Ann Taylor, J. Crew, Ralph Lauren, Sears—it didn't matter who. The point was to utilize the closed system and let someone else's paid, trained design team manage Column 2, eliminating the possibility of errors. It would be like copying a speech from a book instead of coming up with your own. "If you just always wore their stuff, all the time," he reasoned, "you'd always look reasonably good."

It did make a certain sense to leave the aesthetics to the Aubreys of the world and spend my own energy on something else. The single-retailer strategy was the fashionista version of donning a uniform, and had I adopted it, I would have avoided a hundred appearance train wrecks, including the outfit I considered my single worst ever: knee-high brown suede boots, shiny white tights, and a khaki miniskirt overall thing with a denim shirt underneath. Even though I sensed this outfit was a failure, I wore it optimistically several times in the winter of 1998. In it, I imagined myself tripping gaily through the ice-sparkled streets of New York, reading in my bohemian apartment share, laughing with friends at a hip downtown bar. There was something I really wanted to say with this outfit, something that no one else was saying, or had said.

With good reason. According to the chart, that outfit failed in all three columns.

This was true. The boots were uncomfortable relics from eighth grade and had no traction on ice. The miniskirt barely passed as office wear, and the good friends were laughing their asses off about the super-pointed collar on that denim shirt. If I'd been expressing some personal style or identity, it was not very cogent.

I'll take a stab here. "Sexually liberated Annie Oakley takes Manhattan. On a shoestring."

Yeah. That was it.

As I sat tapping my pencil against my chart that night, I understood exactly why that outfit was bad. What I didn't understand was why I stood by it. But I did.

NOT LONG AFTER I MADE MY CHART, HATTIE AND I HAD A PLAYDATE with Anne and Eva upstairs. Anne did not ever seem to have fashion struggles. She had an unerring sense of what was appropriate, knew what looked good on her, and did not bother with anything else. She also researched her purchases—sometimes to a degree I found astounding. Would I ever bother to browse several online children's catalogs for a nice pair of pants for Hattie? No. I would go to the open-air market in Stanley, buy fifteen half-priced items in the span of an hour, and end up not using three or four because they were the wrong size or had a flaw I'd not spotted in my haste.

This waste never happened to Anne, and she always seemed to end up with things that were both beautiful and useful, like her leather bag. It was plain, quilted leather and looked just as good carrying baby snacks as it did over her shoulder when she went out for a hairdo and lunch. I, on the other hand, had recently bagged up ten pleather, cloth, or bead purses that were too small, too big, nonfunctional, out-of-date, or ugly.

While the little girls pattered up and down Anne's hall pulling roller toys, she and I sat on the smooth, cool floor of her apartment, eating squares of chocolate, and bemoaning the pollution and unseasonable heat. I still longed to tell her about my experiment, but as always, I worried how she would feel afterward, telling me about a new purchase. Instead, I asked how *she* would go about buying a nice leather handbag, one that could occasionally stand in for my diaper-and-snacks backpack.

"You should go down to Harvey Nics or Lane Crawford and see what they have," she said. "Try them out."

"Isn't Harvey Nichols really expensive?"

"It's not so bad if you look around," she said. "They've got a big selection, so you can see what you like. Better to get a decent one, anyway, than some tat from the lanes that's going to fall apart in three months."

The idea softened and dispersed delectably through my mind as if it were some of the chocolate we were eating. If I was going to take the trouble to get something, I should think about it, I should really like it, it should be a good one, and it should last.

Yum.

The next time John was home on a weekend, I went out to Harvey Nichols but left the credit card behind. Wide-eyed, I immersed myself in its polished universe of chrome, ingratiating saleswomen, and radically effective facial creams. In accessories, there were handbags with tassels and gold clasps. There were handbags with croc skin and ostrich. There were short handles and long straps and—aha. Convertibles. You could hold the thing by handles, or utilize a secretly tucked-away shoulder strap. I made a note. I was doing research, not shopping, so why not bring a notebook? Handbags segued into sunglasses. I tried on about seven pairs, one of them lovingly placed on a yellow silk pillow for me to retrieve.

"Shall I ring these up for you?" my attentive helper crooned.

"No, thank you," I crooned back, and we both smiled.

I spent a calm, enjoyable hour in Harvey Nichols, untroubled by the possibility of owning anything. I was as detached as if I were in a library or museum, and from this distance I didn't see much I liked.

You should try Joyce.

I'd thought I'd left the Voice at home with my credit card.

Go over to Joyce, she insisted.

There were many stores hawking couture in Hong Kong, but Joyce's massive flagship store dominated Queen's Road.

It was unclear who Joyce was, but her wacky advertisements were plastered in every bus stop around the city—women sitting on alligators or trapped in giant vases like distraught flowers.* On impulse, I left Harvey Nichols and walked the half block to Joyce. A doorman swung the glass panels wide for me, and I entered a lobby dominated by a fifteen-foot statue whose ball gown was composed of roots, twigs, peacock feathers, navy silk, telephones, salad forks, printed scarves, and other effluvia. Instead of a head, there was a rack of elk horns.

See?

After so many months of wearing gray underwear and sporting unmasked blemishes, I walked around Joyce's shrine to sartorial beauty with my hands clasped carefully behind my back. My eyes smarted as I stared at the stitching details on a leather jacket and the strange glossy pyramid of a bag. It was more art gallery than store, with the merchandise on pedestals and under glass. Reverently, I climbed a set of white stairs to the second level to see the gowns. They hung three to a wall, like giant birds at rest, and when I reached out and touched the nearest one—lavender-gray chiffon—I felt a preadolescent sizzle of desire. Layers of scalloped mist cascaded to the floor. The bodice must have been a masterpiece of pleating, padding, and invisible boning, but it looked as if it were simply a piece of silk blown across a female torso by the wind.

Try it.

I glanced around in search of a dressing room.

You can try it on.

You can pretend.

---

* Joyce Ma founded her fashion import company in 1970. She remains so omnipresent in Hong Kong that someone named a bar after her, sort of. It's a tiny hole-in-the-wall with an open-mic night called "Joyce Is Not Here." I never went, but wish I had.

Pretend. The word shot my feathered hope right out of the sky. When would I ever, in my whole life, get to wear such a dress for real? Was I still expecting my invitation to the Costume Institute Gala or the Venice Carnivale to show up in the mail? Detachment became a stern parent dishing out tough love. Delight, then desire, then despair. This was how I got worked over, every single time. I brushed the pale fabric with my knuckles, masochistically searching for a price tag. There was none, proving that whatever beauty Joyce was offering, it was not being offered to me. When I heard the stilettos of an approaching saleswoman, I dropped the hem of the gown and fled.

On my way home, I stared out the window of the bus at the old ladies in their floral pajamas, the salarymen in their dark suits, and the teenage girls in their tidy burgundy-and-gray school uniforms. I understood these garments, but I'd been the kid who dressed as Malificent the Evil for Halloween, whose favorite prom dress was covered in giant blue sequins. When shopping for a wedding dress, I'd sought out the most elaborate gold-and-white, multilayered, off-the-shoulder, hoop-skirted monstrosity in David's Bridal, put it on, and twirled around. What I bought was less flamboyant, but still costumey: a turn-of-the-century tea dress that would have been just as at home on the *Titanic* as on the porch of the Victorian house where we got married. And now? There was none of this flamboyant aspect of myself left in my daily roles as mother and wife: no play, no make-pretend, no drama. If fashion was a language I spoke badly, I also spoke mostly in prose. No songs, no poems—my life during the experiment read more like newspaper text.

That night as I lay in bed, I thought about how my grandmother's sense of fashion had been shaped by climbing out of one world into another she thought was more important. My mother's had been shaped by leaving a known world behind.

My own fashion sense had been shaped by seventeen ZIP codes before I was thirty and, more recently, living on three continents. It was no wonder I felt like a woman lost in translation, my closet a scrap heap of identities, and the song of myself a garbled mess. Even if every human spoke the language of clothes, it was not an Esperanto. Nuances of local dialect were tricky and could take years to get right. I did with fashion what I did with every language I spoke badly. A friend in Cameroon had even given me the word for what I did: *Je débrouiller.* I managed.

This was why I stood by the Annie Oakley outfit, I realized, and why, in some regards, I stood by the flaming-red holiday dress with its giant theatrical sleeves. In every language, I was a winger, an improviser, an actress, and a clown, and for most of my life I'd been proud of that. As an artist of my own life, I frequently let the grammar go to hell, believing rules were made to clarify expression, not shut it down. By aiming too narrowly at perfectly appropriate, I'd ended up with my experiment: an angry anti-art project of the self, a black-and-white photo of a rainbow.

I got up out of bed and went over to my pile of black plastic garbage bags. I ripped one open and dug out the butterfly muumuu I'd packed away. I pulled out some odd red pants,

Survey Question

It might be said that a woman's face, figure, and wardrobe are her most important art project. How do you feel about this statement?

I agree	3%
I agree somewhat	44%
I don't agree	44%
Other	7%

the practical thrift-store raincoat, and the golden scarf. I put all these sides of myself back in my wardrobe between the worn-out momwear and the good-as-new red dress.

The next day I took everything else to the donation bin.

Snapshot: *Artist and Archaeologist*

BOSTON, OCTOBER 30, 2011

What's most impressive about my castoffs—the many I made that day and the fewer I make now—is their volume. A thousand years ago, trends in clothing were pegged to political or religious regimes and changed every few hundred years. Today, mass-produced garments and global distribution networks have melted this slow-moving glacier of taste into a tsunami that has six retail seasons, a two-week runway-to-sales rack turnaround, an average 300 percent retail markup, and a legion of people with box cutters standing by to destroy proprietary overstock. In such a climate, it's no surprise the unsuspecting life-artist-in-all-of-us gets overwhelmed by this flood of garments, nearly drowns in the choices, and then gets washed up on a bleak shore alongside sixty tons per day of outdated, poorly made, or simply unwanted clothes.*

If half of me is that life-artist, the other half is archaeologist, digging through those plastic bags I leave for Goodwill. Today, I know what I didn't during my experiment: that packed in those bags are usually garments made out of questionable fabrics and sewn in less-than-ideal conditions.

* Some 29 million pounds of textile clothing were donated to Goodwill in 2009, including 800,000 pounds of shoes and 285,000 pounds of purses.

Whereas some of those garments will be sold in the United States to fund good works, most of them will end up in the giant warehouses of secondhand clothes dealers who ship them to markets in Asia and Africa. There they may bolster local trade, but they'll also sap the livelihood of indigenous textile workers.

Seeing myself in the context of this tidal wave has helped me work out some new rules for the way I use and buy clothes. First and foremost, I've traded in someone else's must-have list in favor of my own. The taste mavens may wince, but I'm a big fan of the skort and culotte; functional pocketry; performance fabrics; hot shoes that factor in traction, arch support, and low heels; and swimsuits that support me in my decision not to sweat the bikini-hairline maintenance. (These last are incredibly hard to find.)

Second, I've worked out some shopping guidelines for myself, and I use them whenever I make a purchase—my new winter coat, for example. Today, my first rule of shopping is to *Know Exactly What I Want.* Before I got anywhere near a store this fall, I'd already worked out what this coat needed to have or do in all three columns of my chart: gripper cuffs, 650 down fill, removable hood (Column 1); be a neutral color and not make me look like an inflatable character (Column 2); and not be black, charcoal, dark green, midnight purple, or any other color that made me feel like crawling back into bed on a subzero morning (Column 3). My second rule is *Shop Twice.* At the discount store, I tried on twenty coats and bought none. I went home and shopped online, comparing. Later in the week, I hit a sporting-goods store and zeroed in on a pretty pale-beige coat that hadn't even made it out onto the sales floor yet. I tried it on, left it, did other winterwear shopping, and came back later to inspect it more closely because my third rule of shopping is the *Seven-Year Rule.* My most beloved garments have lasted at least that long, and if a new purchase isn't up to that standard, it goes back on the rack.

At the store, I put the coat on a second time and did a few jumping jacks to see how it moved. The thing felt like a cloud with a velvet lining and heated up like a woodstove. It was a reputable brand from a store that was worker friendly, promoted sustainable manufacturing practices, and had a great return policy. It was expensive—almost as expensive as the red dress. But if I wore it every day between November and April for seven years, it worked out to only a few cents per wear—a luxury of comfort and function far less costly than the onetime cash dump of that red dress. It seemed like a really well-thought-out and practical purchase until I zipped it all the way up. The silky fake fur of the hood framed my face and transported me to the steppes outside St. Petersburg where I was a czarina traveling by sleigh to my dacha. Rule number four: *Love It.*

It is not a perfect coat. The day after I bought it I wondered if I should have gotten a vintage winter coat for half the price, and a week later I got the arms tailored because they were a tad puffy.* But after that I forgot it—the whole shopping process of needing, considering, selecting, reconsidering, and adjusting. My final rule of shopping and getting dressed is to remember that *I Do Not (Want to) Live in a Catalog World* because there wouldn't be room in it for me—at least not in costume.

---

*I even went to a secondhand store to try on a few old coats, but they felt like lead aprons. I do strive for compassionate consumption; I get things repaired, remade, and tailored and buy gently used, fair trade, and organic whenever possible, but a nitpicky attention to this stuff puts too much responsibility on me, I feel, and not enough on a textile and garment industry that could stand improvement.

It's Halloween, and five-year-old Hattie and I are getting ready for our first annual pumpkin-carving party. I hull the strawberries while she goes off to arrange and rearrange the napkins in fan patterns, tape her hand-lettered menu on the wall, and sort the gift pencils into scary patterns and cute patterns. I did not make her this way, I swear. I talked her out of dresses when it was cold, I cut her hair short, and I gave her trucks, Legos, and astronaut suits to dress up in—and some of it took—but when the alarm on my phone goes off this Halloween morning, she shouts, "Mama, it's time," and rushes up to her room to don a voluminous pink-tulle dress. She is Glinda the Good Witch from *The Wizard of Oz* this morning, with an aluminum-foil crown and a starry wand she bedazzled herself.

When Hattie comes downstairs in her Glinda outfit, she sees me dressed up in my two-foot-tall purple-feather headdress, bleeding-red lipstick, and every bead necklace I own. "Mama Voulababasse!" she cheers.

She knows the name of the character I am playing because I am the same freaky, pan-cultural spook I played last year—and invented the year before. I felt her beginning to bubble up in middle October when the first pumpkins appeared on porches, and I started wondering where I could get a necklace made of bones. One of the greatest surprises of parenting has been my own opportunity to wear belted leotards and do accents and silly walks. One day much too soon this will mortify my children, but by then, I hope, I'll have the time to try out for community theater. It's not the Venice Carnivale, but it's what I have on hand.

As I set out our freaky fruit salad and deep-fried eyeballs for this party, the trickster in me reflects. Costumes allow a wearer extraordinary freedoms. She gets to be who she ordinarily is not, but also to notice who she ordinarily is. In a way, my experiment was a bit like wearing an outlandish feather headdress for a year—it felt thrilling and a little dangerous to play the part at first. In the final months, though, when the artifice became familiar, I began to question all the ready-made, one-size-fits-all garments of the self I usually put on, not realizing the subtler dangers in these daily roles, how much these sometimes cost me, or who else I was asking to pay.

The Empty Jar

Most women are one man away from welfare.

—GLORIA STEINEM, AMERICAN FEMINIST, JOURNALIST, AND POLITICAL ACTIVIST

HONG KONG, DECEMBER 2007

One winter night, standing in our tiny Hong Kong kitchen over a pile of dirty dishes, I turned off the water and let my hands fall limp. John was out of town as usual, Hattie was finally asleep, and in my mind I'd been singing my song of anger as I scraped and sudsed: there was despair over the inequity of domestic duties, frustration about all the work travel, and fury about John's time-management skills. I hadn't signed up to be a single parent. Working through these verses had become my dark and private hobby, and most nights now, they supplanted any thoughts about my experiment.

But the Christmas holiday was coming. We were going to Australia to visit John's sister and her family. We'd be together for two weeks without interruption. It was everything I wanted, yet I felt my anger pressing against this potential for happiness like a storm-swelled reservoir behind a rotted dam. *I can't do it,* I thought, mashing the soap bubbles in the sink. If, in my current state of mind, I had to play "Happywife" for two weeks straight in Australia, the dam would surely break. The flood would be ugly, bad, and poorly timed. A good wife and mother—a good *person*—would never let her own mood ruin anyone else's Christmas.

You need to start taking care of yourself, the Voice said. *Since someone else is never around to help do the job.*

I'd had a conversation with my friend Corinne recently, as she'd given me and Hattie a lift to a playgroup outing. I'd been singing my angry song to her when she cut me off. "It's not John's job that's the problem," she pointed out. "It's your quality of life. You're not having enough fun," she declared. "If you were taking better care of yourself, you wouldn't be bothered by him. You could be happy and supportive."

My response to this accusation was extreme—a sudden, authentic coughing fit so violent that Corinne asked if she needed to stop the car. I said no, cleared the bitter self-recognition that was choking me, settled back into the seat, and cracked open one of the diet Cokes Corinne kept chilled in the glove compartment.

Corinne was not a show-off, and never vain. She *did* happen to be quite good at taking care of herself—a habit that was necessary, she felt, if she was going to put up with a husband who traveled even more than John. She also had a young family, but her approach to managing the household was opposite mine. She was not slogging through chores and logistics on her own. She was getting help from amahs; from her mother, who flew over several times a year; and from a local preschool. She was a terrific and involved mom, but also constantly booking trips, hosting gatherings, and connecting people with each other. And when it all got to be too much, she didn't beat her head against a wall or skewer her husband with angry looks during their brief time together; she simply headed for the spa.

Go book it right now.

I shucked off the dish-washing gloves and went into the office. I flipped through the file cabinet beside the desk until I found the golden folder. It was only a yellow plastic sleeve, but in it were my treasures: a coupon for free mango pudding at a favorite dessert spot and the AsiaMiles reward catalog. There was also one thick cream envelope that drastically outclassed all the rest. It was a gift certificate to the Peninsula Hotel—its restaurants, gift shop, or spa—given by a generous cousin who often passed through Hong Kong on business. This luxury I had been hoarding for eleven months, waiting to use it for a nice dinner out with John. Now there were only three weeks before it expired.

I did not waffle about whether I would be violating the experiment's rules or whether John could take Hattie when he was still jet-lagged. I simply picked up my phone and dialed.

"How can I help you?" said an unhurried, honeyed female voice. I could smell the clean sheets and fresh flowers through the phone. The Voice inside me purred as this other one advised me to pull up the online spa menu so she could guide me though the list of delights. She helped me settle on a total pampering package that would consume the gift certificate.

"Will there be anything else this evening, ma'am?"

There would not. The Peninsula phone angel and I parted ways but not before she told me how much she was looking forward to my visit. Disingenuous it might have been, but wow, did it make me feel great.

I also knew that the equation of money for good feelings was not so simple. Two feet from where I sat making that end-of-my-rope call was the clear-plastic flip-top container: my experiment's philanthropy jar. The notebook with various material cravings was still in there, although as the months went on, the entries had gotten fewer. The money for the jeans I hadn't bought and for the swimsuit I had bought was in there. The rest of the contributions I'd made were gone, frittered away on bus fare and runs to the grocery because our bank was inconvenient and I was always cash poor.

The jar's emptiness bothered me. My selfishness, stinginess, and greed bothered me. To absolve myself, I'd tried to imagine cutting a big check at the end—I could probably guess at an approximate amount—but when I did this, I didn't see a benevolent woman handing money out to make the world a better place; I saw a dependent wife needling her breadwinning elephant husband, and possibly getting gored because of it.

I still wanted to believe I could do what I'd set out to do as part of the experiment—feel economically secure enough to share. I wanted to believe it the way I wanted to believe that one day John would call his work done and come home at five. Nearly a year into examining my beliefs, however, I knew them to deviate from reality.

After I made my spa appointment that night, I spent an hour reading couples-counselor bios online and writing down phone numbers to call. As for the jar, it still just sat there, doing no good for anyone.

ON THE DAY OF MY SPA BOOKING, I TOOK THE STAR FERRY ACROSS the harbor to Kowloon. It was a quick ride, but enjoyable because Hong Kong's maritime heritage is better preserved than its architectural one: fifties-era boats bobbed directly in the shadow of towering skyscrapers. We passengers filed into quaint wooden benches along open-air decks while crewmen in white-and-blue sailor's tunics tossed the giant mooring lines aboard. Technically, a spa visit *had* to be classed as beauty spending, I thought, as I found a spot near the edge where I could feel the salt spray. Yet my experiment would mean nothing if I did not come out of it sane. This was less a verboten beauty indulgence than a wise and personally therapeutic act, I rationalized. Plus, the thing was about to expire!

It was hard to think "therapy," however, as I strolled through the Peninsula's lofty marble lobby. It was even harder when I was ushered into a treatment room and my foot ceremony began. A clinician pored elixirs over my feet—hot, cold, scented, oily—and left me alone to soak in a bucket of flower petals. Luxury it was, and I tried to get into it, but really I just felt embarrassed for the woman who had to kneel down before me and deal with my archless, calloused lumps of clay.

Next came a sweat in the superheated crystal sauna, followed by a massage so gently powerful that my anger and sadness burst through the dam. My masseuse calmly handed me tissues as I cried right there on the padded table, naked under my towel. When the flood subsided, I wondered how often, in such deluxe establishments, the staff witnessed patron breakdowns. Some smidgen of allegiance to my experiment—combined with a growing distaste for beauty treatments involving pain—had kept me from booking a facial, so when I'd finished sniffling, I wrapped myself in a bathrobe and headed for the luxury of all luxuries—the nap room.

I stood at the entrance of a sunny, quiet chamber filled with polished teak and lofty white chaise lounges. Near the door, a table was spread with teas, water, green apples, and a stack of beauty and fashion magazines. I thought: the staff of the Peninsula has done so much work to banish my worries, why read a whole book full of more? Then again, the first time I'd encountered a nap room in a spa, I'd thought to myself: why not just sleep at home? I hadn't been able to imagine a home that was a workplace filled with duties, not a quiet sanctuary. Today, my foot ceremony had been similarly lost on me, probably because I never wore high heels and didn't have to stand up for hours a day. The definition of luxury, I realized, was as relative as the definition of beauty. When a woman entered behind me and picked up a magazine, I smiled at her.

If everyone had different spa needs, I thought, padding over to one of the chaise lounges, the need itself we seemed to have in common. The nap room was packed with women in robes and head towels reclining, murmuring to each other, sleeping with arms luxuriously outstretched. After my big cry, this scene of women arrayed in attitudes of repose was bittersweet. Here was womanhood tired and spent; here was beauty wounded. Without makeup or jewelry, and dressed in identical white terry cloth, our differences in age, taste, profession, and status were mostly erased.

Survey Question

Which of the following are pressing concerns of yours right now?

	Women	Men
General physical and mental health	71%	57%
Money	61%	66%
Job or school	59%	59%
Gender-specific health issues	17%	10%

As I sank into the marshmallowy cushion, I felt a jag of tenderness toward each of these women. Just like me, they'd come to take refuge in warm steam, massage, hot rocks, skin scrubs, or this quiet, pillowed room. What anger, stress, sadness, fatigue, or boredom had brought each of them here? What were their stories?

Well, maybe that one near the window has a new baby. The girls up front might be celebrating a birthday, or mourning a breakup. Maybe the one wearing the toe separators just kicked cancer, or landed a big client.

I'd been noticing a change in my inner Voice. She was softer and less judgmental—of me and the women around me. As a result, I wasn't fighting her as much. The shift had begun after that birthday party with Aubrey, when I was forced to admit there were some good reasons for the bad habits my inner Voice espoused. And now the nap room. I could no more argue with these women's need to be here than with the inner Voice that had sent me along, too.

And yet, I knew this deluxe self-care strategy had serious drawbacks. In two hours I would open the door to a husband frantically sending work e-mails and a hungry kid with a soaked diaper. Tension would instantly knot up my shoulders and stay there for the next three years until I had another blessed excuse to visit a spa. The spa was great when you (or your cousin) could spring for it, but its effects were short-lived. It was a Band-Aid, not a solution.

You're still here, aren't you?

Sometimes, my inner Voice seemed to be wiser to my female reality than I was. I understood now she was just trying to be on my side—even when I insisted I did not like to take sides. It would have been nice, in the warm, quiet nap room, if my inner Voice *had* been a real person beside me. A girlfriend even, who'd shared the challenges of the past months and who'd felt the release of the cry and the massage as keenly as I had. If my inner Voice had been lying on the chaise lounge next to mine, wrapped in her own white Turkish terry-cloth robe, I could have turned to her and asked, "Why do we all feel we have to get away from our own lives?"

I think she would have looked up from her beauty magazine—spacers on her toes to protect the pedi, some toxic blue paste on her face—and asked her own question in return: *What else can we do?*

I sighed, sank deeper into my chaise, and folded my own unmanicured mitts across my belly. The nap room's wooden shutters broke the afternoon light into gold rays across my legs. Like good sex, or a good workout, the good spa visit brought on an afterglow of clarity. I did feel healed now, somewhat. I also knew that what wounded me most deeply was my anger.

"I AM FURIOUS AND HURT," I TOLD THE THERAPIST THE FOLLOWING weekend. "And desperate to change that before next Tuesday." I'd booked myself an appointment with a relationship counselor and arrived with a three-page manifesto of grievances copied straight from my cherished song of rage. Once I started singing my blues, I couldn't stop—I was disappointed, I was confused, and I felt unappreciated. I was a therapist's thesaurus of bad feelings and worse behavior, which I had absolutely no trouble at all articulating, providing examples for, and elaborating on if, for any reason, he wasn't getting the picture. I was fighting a thousand battles every day but doing it in a vat of Jell-O—resistance to my best efforts was high on every side, and nothing I did made any headway! Worse, my own husband was too busy to give a shit.

The therapist gave a good show of giving one—pencil in mouth, nodding, murmuring *I see*—and for this reason, my rant could have run into the "multiple-hour therapy intensive" category on his price chart if my phone hadn't rung.

The first time, I ignored it. When the phone rang again, I picked up and found it was the secretary at Joni and Kai, calling to remind me of my hair appointment in fifteen minutes. After the spa visit, I'd decided that things would go better in Australia if I got a trim. And if I was going to break all my experiment's rules this week and do beauty self-care, I might as well get that trim at a place familiar with Western hair—namely, one of the trendiest salons in downtown Hong Kong. I hung up and told the therapist about the fifteen minutes.

"I'm sure they'll save your appointment if you're a little late," the therapist said.

We went on for another fifteen minutes.

"I'm sure you're right," I said, "but let me just call them and let them know."

He waited patiently while I called.

It was in the middle of this second call that I saw myself as that unknown therapist must have seen me that day—frenzied equally with anger and with hair maintenance, organizing my time around a salon visit and a vacation. This wasn't me, was it? There were boundaries here that were blurred. The self was trying to make a stand . . . by sitting down in a stylist's chair? I would solve my marital problems with . . . pampering? When I hung up my phone, I told the therapist about my experiment, as an excuse or counterpoint to my behavior. He just bit his pencil and nodded. His closing words to me were this:

"You seem to want someone to tell you you're doing a good job with all of this. You are. It's a good thing you came to see me, and I think it's good that you're being open with your husband."

As I trotted over to my appointment, the Voice added, *And it's a good thing you're taking care of yourself.*

But the confidence I'd placed in my self-care strategy was wavering, and it wavered further at Joni and Kai. Because I'd made the salon wait, the salon made me wait. When it was finally my turn, the shampooist tossed a gown at me and gave me a splashy, lukewarm hair wash while chatting with her compatriot at the next sink. My stylist, when he arrived, spent just over three minutes combing and snipping my hair before he went over to kibitz with another client.

It's just because you're not a regular, the Voice explained.

I understood, but then he did it again. He asked about the shape of the cut long after he could have done anything about it. I could have complained, but part of me wasn't ready to offend a person using scissors near my eyes. The other part was curious about how far he would go. He went further than I could have imagined: between the cut and the blow-dry, he went and got himself a cup of tea. (Perhaps he was testing how far *I* would go?) The bill for the privilege of being ignored for nearly an hour came to $700 HK, or $87.50 US. This was roughly $50 more than my last cut at Squiffy, a haircut that was just as mediocre and included a brief shoulder massage for the price.

Survey Questions

How often do you feel suckered or pushed into buying something you later don't like or need?

Often	3%
Occasionally	29%
Rarely	53%
Never	13%

How often do you feel guilty about something you've bought, either because it's frivolous, too expensive, not quite in line with your values (or your partner's values), or not worth what you paid?

Often	7%
Occasionally	39%
Rarely	48%
Never	4%

This is why, I thought to myself, standing at the front counter, jostled by other women waiting to be overcharged and neglected. THIS. IS. WHY. I put it on the credit card and went home. If John noticed the haircut, he said nothing about it, and I sure didn't ask.

I knew, of course, that John was going to see the charge, and days later, he did.

"Who is Joni and Kai?" he asked. "What did I pay them $700 for?" (He wasn't doing it on purpose, but the Hong Kong currency made the question sound so much worse.)

Despite being ready for this inquisition, I froze, paralyzed by my choices. I could (a) tell the truth about how bad the haircut had been, and then wallow in self-loathing. Alternately, I could (b) ignore my own beef with Joni and Kai and their stylist, Asshole Sassoon, and cast the haircut as a proactive, if expensive, effort to take care of myself.

I chose (b) but didn't like it. I felt myself joining a long, underhanded female tradition of paying myself for efforts no one else seemed to value. I could have exacted this self-care/self-payment in any number of ways, but like many women, I reflexively reached for beauty: new clothes, new flats, spa packages, hair care, luxury domestic goods. "I am working so hard and doing so much and not getting anything for it," went the thinking, "so I am forced to give it to myself." Beauty-revenge spending, it might be called, a passive aggression and survival technique.

The undervalued woman's song of anger was an old one—I'd heard other women singing it, probably ever since money replaced female-friendly economic traditions like bartering, labor swapping, and communal land stewardship.* When I sang it to my girlfriends, they often added verses of their own, so I felt as if I was part of a great chorus. But that night, as I stood in the kitchen door, clucking and fussing, and John sat hunched over his computer, scowling and sad, I realized that

* To hear a catchy contemporary rendition of this song of anger, check out Blue Cantrell's "Hit 'Em Up Style" in which a woman spends all her cheating husband's cash at Neiman Marcus and then sells his house and car.

all my loud notes of hurt had a counterpart in John's wordless, pinched stoicism.

This pain wasn't a solo; it was a duet.

Snapshot: *A New Accounting*

Boston, November 2011

When I finally noticed the emptiness of my experiment's philanthropy jar, it came as an unpleasant surprise, but perhaps it shouldn't have. Without realizing when, how, or why it happened, I'd become one of the 90 percent of women who felt financially insecure, whether because they spent unwisely, chronically underinvested in their retirement funds, were paid less than men, fell into old family patterns, or performed caretaking or other work that has long been undervalued in a monetary economy. It's not all of us, certainly, and studies show that younger women ages twenty-five to thirty-four tend to spend as much as men and are just as savvy with their stock picks.

Survey Question

Please rate your financial independence.

	Women	Men
Completely independent	28%	48%
Completely dependent	14%	1%

Unfortunately, that hadn't been me. Because John had studied finance, and because I'd always earned a fraction of what he did, I had been glad to hand the financial reins over early in our marriage. Five years in, though, this plan was backfiring. John felt like a slave to his work, lavishing all his time on it. I felt like a slave to John's financial anxiety and rebelled with bipolar money habits: I could outscrimp him with my experiment or pay myself reparations with beauty revenges like the red dress and the spa. Either way, that moment of marital accounting during my experiment—John checking the credit-card statement and finding it inflated, me checking my emotional balance and finding myself falling far short—was a watershed moment, one in which I realized that an antiquated marital accounting between husband and wife was costing us both too much.

In the years since, I've realized I wasn't alone in salving my anger and frustration with material happiness. Many of my own survey respondents felt a link between beauty spending and other anxieties. A different survey (not mine) asked working mothers how they relieved stress. The number-one strategy was exercise, and the number-two strategy was shopping. I've begun to think a culturally sanctioned habit of retail therapy in the world's wealthiest, more educated women is a little like the behavior of men in impoverished countries. In some studies, these men have been shown to be more likely than their female counterparts to drink, smoke, gamble, or otherwise fritter their resources away. It's a case of feeling only half-empowered: poor men and moderately wealthy women have some power (power over the day's earnings, power over their own pleasures) but not nearly enough to remake a system that does them few favors. If the beauty industry has an annual revenue of $10 billion, it feels safe to say that a sizable portion is spent by women not trying to look good, but to escape feeling bad.

Survey Questions

Do you think you spend more money on your appearance (buying clothes, shoes or makeup, getting salon or cosmetic treatments) when you feel anxious, sad, or frustrated in other realms of your life?

Yes	46%
No	53%

Do you think you do more beauty "work" (exercising, dieting, plucking your chin, hemming all your pants, shopping for something hard to find online, organizing your closets) when you feel anxious, sad, or frustrated in other realms of your life?

Yes	39%
No	60%

I needed that cycle to end. I felt needy when I clearly wasn't; I felt shortchanged when I had so much. So last spring I decided to measure just how much I really did have in my own beauty trousseau: the clothes, the personal products, and jewelry. I wrote out a questionnaire I called the "Beauty Wealth Calculator" and then went to my closet and filled it in for myself, hauling out all my pairs of shoes and pairs of jeans and belts and scarves, counting each one, assigning values, adding it all up.* When I got my number, I was shocked. My total beauty wealth was $17,145. Could I really have that much of this stuff? Instead of making me feel guilty, as I'd feared, I felt empowered,

* This Beauty Wealth calculator is available to use on my website, www.phoebebakerhyde.com.

even *personally* wealthy, something I'd never felt, despite living in a household with a comfortable income. I also realized it was real wealth, and therefore something I wanted to take good care of and use wisely, not disparage as junk, feel guilty about, or hoard for some future life I wasn't actually leading.

Survey Question

Overall, which best characterizes how you feel?

I don't feel materially wealthy, but I do feel rich in other ways	53%
I feel materially wealthy and rich in other ways, too	37%
I feel materially wealthy but not rich in other ways	4%
I don't feel materially wealthy, nor do I feel rich in other ways	4%

If my experiment and my survey helped me see how the time, energy, and money women spend on appearance contribute in remarkable ways to happiness and self-worth, getting a dollar figure helped me put that appearance spending in context. I held many emotional and concrete assets in shoes I did not wear, but fewer in other realms of my life—those personal savings and retirement funds I'd let slide, for one, my philanthropy, for another.

Since the end of my experiment, I've drawn up a new balance sheet for myself, both inside of and apart from my marriage. I've reinstated personal checking and retirement accounts that got folded into the pot when John and I bought our first home. I've made spending decisions that reflect how much I value both my roles as a parent and a writer, decisions that John didn't always agree with. I've worked my way toward financial literacy and have even done my own online philanthropic investing. I've also changed my approach to self-care. I still love a massage and a hot soak, but I've realized my spa visit in Hong Kong was a Band-Aid measure for a harried, lonely parent. I will be forever grateful to my friends around the world—and to a savvy pack of women writing do-it-yourself manuals for modern womanhood—for showing me how to share and be shared with, how to more equitably divvy up the labor of child care and household management, and how to look past my Norman Rockwell image of nuclear family life to other open hearts and helping hands all around me. Parenthood, coupledom, and financial partnership are in flux as much today as the men and women in these roles. After almost nine years of marriage, John and I have begun to talk more openly about the gender roles and expectations we bring to our multicultural marriage,* and while this is hard, daily work, I now know that a difference between us needn't end in a silent capitulation to misunderstanding. Instead, it can be a catalyst for growth.

IT IS NINE O'CLOCK ON THURSDAY NIGHT IN BOSTON. JOHN AND I are sitting in our living room having a different disagreement over money. This time it's about bathroom renovations. The one drawback of our new home is baths with peeling wallpaper, a faucet with cold water only, cabinets missing doors, and

* For example, I'm the first woman on either side of my family to keep my maiden name and possibly the first in many generations to work at a career through my children's babyhood. John thinks it's a lot of fuss over nothing: traditionally Chinese women keep their names, and his mother brought home a paycheck every week of his life—with the help of live-at-home grandparents.

an unusable shower filled with broken tile. In the past two months, I've made drawings, visited overstock websites, and talked options with two different contractors about how to minimize costs. John is sitting in a rocker as I explain all this.

"Okay, okay, okay," he says. "Just give me the numbers."

I do. The two contractors' estimates are virtually the same.

"That's three times what we estimated," John says.

"Yeah," I say, "we had no idea what this was going to cost us."

John counts out our savings and assets on his fingers for me. "It's going to take a big chunk of savings, and that's not easy to replace," he says. "You don't want to be house poor, because what if something happens?"

"I know."

"Can't you ask them to bring it down? Or deal with someone else? I know we're heading into construction season, but come on."

I stare down at the ideas and calculations spread across my lap. John is rocking with a tight, anxious expression on his face and tapping his pen against the rocker's arm. We bought that rocker at a flea market for ten bucks when we were first married. I nursed both kids in it, even though the bare wood armrests cut into my forearms. Back then, I lacked the energy to wrap the arms in dishtowels or get them padded, and John never did it for me because he never sat in the chair. Also, I never asked.

I leaf thoughtfully through my papers. "Maybe we can just fix the plumbing and repaint the tile," I say. "There are pictures of how that looks on the Internet. I can probably figure out how to grout. I refinished a dresser once. Or we could use an unlicensed contractor."

"No, it will end up looking terrible," he says, getting up and grabbing his work bag to head upstairs. "Just e-mail them. See what they can change."

This meeting I've been looking forward to all day is over. It took ten minutes.

"Thanks for doing all this," John adds on his way upstairs.

"Yeah," I say, slumped on the couch and motionless with guilt for not being an ace handywoman and for the sin of even *thinking* about depleting our savings. In the context of world suffering, a broken shower is nothing, I tell myself. I should just shove a potted ficus in there and be grateful.

My head is swirling as I put everything away in its file. On my own way up the stairs I realize: bathroom renovations are the new red dress. This is *just* like the overpriced haircut at Joni and Kai. Somehow the same pattern is at work: I ask; John denies. I spend; John scolds. I am afraid to disagree with him and lose his favor; he is afraid to agree with me and lose the favor of the world. I hate this dynamic with all my might, yet I seem powerless to stop it from happening.

But I'm not powerless to notice it, and react differently. I know now—after far more therapy than just that one visit—that I don't have to cave in and cry, or try to beat John at his own game ("Yeah, screw the new bathroom. I don't even *like* hot water that much!"). I also don't have to defend what very well might be high estimates. There's another position here, not John's, not that of the salespeople or service providers, and no longer that of a needy but financially underinformed caregiver. Now there's my own position: conscientious but not timid, well aware of our financial situation, and not afraid to act as a partner in this relationship instead of a disgruntled subordinate scrounging for a lesser payoff. During the last months of my experiment, I might have been going about self-care the wrong way, but I was right about needing it, and I think I'm right on this, too.

I wait for my sulky, "if-I-can't-have-it-my-way-I-don't-want-it" reaction to pass. Maybe one day I'll overcome this emotional reflex, but I'm not there yet. Then, in the days following our conversation, I tell John how much his lack of enthusiasm for my economical design ideas hurt. I need a sounding board for this project, I say, not a "no" man. This label upsets him, and he reminds me that he's said yes to a few things recently—smaller investments of time, attention, and money that feel significant to him. I have to agree, they count. I tell him what I know about home values in the area and show him what I believe we can afford. When I contact the contractors for a second round of negotiation, John thanks me again.

This time, I hear it. And I think: it's fear that so often leaves us feeling empty—fear that causes empty hearts and sometimes empty philanthropy jars as well. Some of us buy diversions and delights, hoping to cheat time and forget death. Others sit on savings forever, budgeting for the imagined wolf at the door. Unfortunately, we'll never know whether these schemes worked to give us better lives—we'll be dead when the results come in. All we can truly assess ourselves is the quality of our daily, hourly, minute-by-minute calculations: how nimbly we count life's riches; how skillfully we fill our emptiness so we may sum to joy.

Outgrowing the Gown

Some day my prince will come / Some day we'll meet again / And away to his castle we'll go / To be happy forever I know.

—SNOW WHITE, STAR OF DISNEY'S 1937 ANIMATED CLASSIC *SNOW WHITE AND THE SEVEN DWARFS*

AUSTRALIA, DECEMBER 2007; HONG KONG, JANUARY 2008

As I prepared for our holiday trip to Australia, I steeled myself for a hard time: distracted husband, disoriented kid. I packed ibuprofen, a fake smile, and novels to hide in. But sometime during the plane ride—probably about the time Hattie fell asleep in John's arms—my anticipatory sulking turned into exhilaration. We were traveling as a family! We were going to a new continent!

It was a terrific shock to land underneath crystalline blue skies after Hong Kong's chronic humidity. Sydney felt architecturally like Great Britain, culturally like Southern California, and vegetatively like nothing I'd ever seen. On our first morning there, John scooped Hattie up and carried her off into one of Sydney's parks so that I could catch up with John's sister, Elaine, who I'd not seen in months.

"So, how is everything with you these days?" she asked as we strolled together down a tidy bricked path, blood-sucking fruit bats hanging in the trees above.

"Well . . . it's been a hard fall," I started. "John has been traveling a lot." Habit caused me to haul out my angry verses, but as I watched John and Hattie running through grass chasing rainbow-colored parrots, my complaints became boring, even to me. Something had sapped my fury of its power; maybe the massage or the counseling session, or that moment of reckoning after the haircut, when I saw my own anxious insecurities mirrored—but different—in John.

It wasn't just John's sister's family we met up with in Australia; it was relatives of theirs as well, plus their three kids. After convening in Sydney, we traveled by van to a big farmhouse in the Blue Mountains, singing and sightseeing. There were a few insects of unusual size in our rented house, but it was surrounded by rolling fields, long-haired goats, and a stream. There was even a giant eucalyptus hung with a rope swing. Because we all shared the grocery shopping, meal preparation, and child minding, the dread I'd grown accustomed to most solo evenings was replaced by companionable conversation. Loneliness was replaced by laughter and evening board games. Grandparents far away sent a bumper crop of Christmas gifts, and there was never a shortage of playmates for the kids.

Each family also had its own unique split-out of duties, and it was refreshing to remember that in other cultures, and other families, it was sometimes the men who remembered the car seats, minced the garlic, and defused the tantrums and the women whose jobs took the family all over the world. Although I'd set out to put on a brave face in Australia, I quickly understood I wasn't being called on to play Happywife—only to be myself, sometimes even before being a parent. I could be the self who *liked* to see new things and take on challenges, who *liked* cooking dinner, who *liked* playing with the kids, who had plenty of time for friends and found it easy, not difficult, to be a good sport.

One lazy afternoon I found John asleep on a couch with a *National Geographic* splayed open on his chest—his accounting literature abandoned on the floor. Here was the real John, not the John of my pissed-off imagination. I had a pang of empathy for him right then. The same thing sometimes happened to me—I'd get stuck in a novel I'd already read when I was supposed to be sanitizing toys, doing dishes, or reading up on potty-training techniques. It wasn't just me who was having trouble adjusting to a new identity; John was dealing with a definition of personhood that was new to him, too.

As I looked at him asleep on the couch in an old band T-shirt and shredded jeans, I was able to remember the kid who'd wooed me with an original song sung in a cut-rate apartment filled with mosquitoes. He took me to jazz sets; he made me mixes; he told me to close my eyes and listen in the dark. He'd had his cello boxed in plywood and shipped across the Pacific because he couldn't bear to think of it in storage, but after those bucolic two weeks of playing it to Hattie during paternity leave, he'd played it only three or four times in more than two years. He'd hoped to improve his Mandarin in Hong Kong and to travel in the Mainland—it was a big part of why we'd even come—but his schedule had conflicted with all the lessons he'd signed up for and the personal travel as well. My goofball, K-mart-loving, ex-band-member husband now had a closet full of custom suits and was expected to dole out money-filled red envelopes at the Chinese New Year like the boss he was. He loved Hattie desperately, but like most babies, Hattie preferred her primary caregiver (me), and her rejections twisted John's face with a pain that I felt, too.

All these things I knew individually, but locked inside my own anger, I'd never seen the picture they made together. The day before we left for Sydney, John had gone to see the couples counselor by himself, because I'd asked him to. He hadn't told me anything about it, but I had faith it had done some good. We'd made it through weeds before and would again.

I also saw Hattie more clearly during that vacation, especially the day our group took a sightseeing jaunt to Three Sisters Gorge. We oohed and aahed over thin, multicolored spires of rock set in a dramatic wooded chasm, and afterward I overcame all my conscientious objections to white sugar and hydrogenated oils and watched Hattie negotiate her first ice cream Drumstick. I saw that she did not rush ahead into chocolate abandon but checked her technique against the rest of us in the rental van chowing down. There was a self-conscious nature at work on the dripping vanilla and unpredictable nuts. Her delight was a private, meticulous, and silent thing, but her quick, dark flares of dislike were loud. She wasn't sold on eating the cone and wouldn't be pushed. At twenty months old, she was already a person with her own perspective and store of knowledge.

One day, I challenged it. No one had tried the rope swing yet, but it looked good to me. The seat was level, and the drop below the branch sufficient. It reminded me of the swings I'd loved as a teen in Vermont when we jumped from a high bank and twirled way out over the freezing Connecticut River. I took hold of the swing, ran toward open air, and flung myself on. Hattie, in John's arms, screamed. The Mama she knew in Hong Kong was extremely cautious. So who was this other woman with the grin, throwing her body around in the air? Hattie cried to see her, and in a moment I stopped. But not before I'd felt that other woman surging back into my body, flooding it with joy.

John's frequent work travel did have one advantage: he had become an airport rock star with points galore. We waited for our return flight in the Qantas business-class lounge.

"Why did that vacation feel more like real life than my real life does?" I asked aloud, not really of John. Hattie was standing behind me on my chair, watching takeoffs through a window. "I guess it's just when you've been away from it for a while," I went on, "this whole thing . . . " I waved my hand around at the leather seats and three-foot flower arrangements, the men in blazers talking into cell phones, the women in pretty blouses tending children with matching suitcases, "it feels weird."

"Just enjoy it," said John, slurping noodles noisily from a bowl. "It won't last."*

He made a good point. Our foreign tour was due to end in a few months, and we would be going somewhere else—possibly back to the States. Although it might be a relief to be back on familiar turf, I didn't want to look back on our time in Hong Kong and remember nothing but fighting: with motherhood, with the expatriate bubble, with my own work, and with the man I loved who just wanted me to be happy.

* Although I didn't know it then, John's comment had far-reaching implications about the expatriate lifestyle, too. Today, his firm no longer sends so many junior employees on overseas tours, instead relying on local staff, or staff who can commit to living in a country permanently. Nongovernmental organizations and global charities have also recognized the downside of plunking outsiders in a foreign culture and are moving toward more equitable models of partnership instead.

"Hey," I said to the top of John's head, "I'm really glad I'm here with you."

He looked up from his bowl. "Me, too," he said, gazing at me with the warm, guileless brown eyes I fell in love with. "Don't you want anything?" he asked plaintively.

"I totally do," I admitted, letting myself sink back into the pillowed lounge chair. "When you go back for thirds, get me one of those tiny little cheeses, please. And a big glass of wine."

He smiled, satisfied. As a philosophy of life, John's wasn't so bad: everyone should fully maximize the complimentary buffet.

IN MID-JANUARY, JOHN BROUGHT HOME THE INVITATION: THE FIRM'S end-of-year party. *True Elegance* was the theme, and the font was thin and looping. No flames this year, but it would again be hundreds of staffers, photo backdrops, and the occasional floor-length gown. Same deal.

I, however, was (or should be) a new woman after eleven months of my experiment. I had learned (or should have learned) many things. One of the most useful was that the definition of beauty depended not only on who was looking but also on what they were looking for. I could change my own focus if I needed to or, if others were looking, pull a sleight of hand. I'd done that very thing recently, when I'd gone to a friend's dressy party wearing a fresh rose behind my ear instead of makeup and jewelry. Picking the rose out with Hattie had been the highlight of my day. It did fall out on the dance floor, but it gave me the boost of appearance self-confidence that the red dress hadn't the year before.

In the days leading up to the firm's party, I began to suspect that the real problem had not been with the red dress or how I looked in it, but with my attitude toward the party itself. I'd been swept up by my own vision of myself, dazzling in a dazzling métier, as red-hot as the font on the invitations in my new dress. And when the whole thing—the party, my outfit, my dazzlement—fell short of my largely self-manufactured hype, the disillusionment was severe. The antidote, then, was to be free of illusions. Maybe the truth was that at my husband's work function, there was really no room for my own red-hotness or true elegance except as an extension of John's status and competence.

"Why don't you pick out my outfit this year?" I suggested to John. "It's your work thing, so maybe I should look the way *you* want me to look. I hereby divest myself of any emotional investment in this party."

He sighed. "Maybe you should give me some options," he said as he stared at his own travel-mangled suits hanging in the closet.

A friend had pressed one of her unneeded cocktail dresses upon me when we were in the States. It was simple and black, so I laid it on the bedspread. Out came the shiny black-patent pumps from last year and a different pair of low black heels I'd bought for a funeral. I didn't pull out any jewelry at first—experiment's rules—but then realized this could be a test. Maybe John didn't even like me in jewelry. Maybe that was all in my head, too. From the back of my wardrobe, I dug out an opera-length set of fake pearls and a demure choker of real ones.

John nodded at the dress. He pointed to the funeral shoes. I bit my tongue. He picked up the short pearl choker.

"You don't think the longer pearls would be more theme-ish?" I asked. "You know, truly elegant Audrey Hepburn?"

"Am I picking, or are you picking?"

I put away the long pearls.

On the day of the party, we both got dressed in under fifteen minutes. After almost a year of hard work, I'd achieved it: true Equivalent Prep Time. While John put on an ordinary work suit and a clean tie, I spent about fifteen seconds checking my reflection in the mirror. I knew my clothes fit me, were clean, and that there were no holes or tears. I brushed my teeth carefully and asked John if I looked presentable. He gave me the all clear, and we left.

"I feel like a conservative senator's wife," I joked as we rode the mirrored elevator downstairs.

He was surprised by my comment, but quiet about it, and seemed to understand that the joy for me, in this outfit, was looking the way he needed me to.

It was a weird party. During the cocktail hour, while young beauties in their Truly Elegant frocks flitted about taking pictures of each other, I stayed wrapped up in a shawl against the polar ventilation system. I quizzed one of John's colleagues about Malaysian sociopolitics and spent a long time at the bar picking out an expensive scotch. At dinner, I swapped mothering war stories with the wives of two partners (warm, approachable, and living lives just like mine) and purposefully faded into the conversational background so I could listen to John talk shop.

What I heard surprised me. John was not in over his head at work—as he so often worried to me; he was, if anything, over *other* people's heads. He was not struggling to earn a smidgen of respect; he was in fine shape. He was kicking ass. It took me by happy surprise between the salad and main course to feel so proud of my own husband. After all, I did love him. I wanted him to do well in things that were important to him.

It felt odd and not entirely comfortable to be the supportive wallflower. But for the first time since arriving in Hong Kong, it felt like something I wanted to do.

John did his socializing and nice-making, and then we drifted out to see the sparkling view of Kowloon from the convention center's lobby.

I took out my camera. "It's been a year," I said. "Almost. This was the party that started my experiment."

"You want me to take a picture of you here?" John asked, confused. "I mean you're dressed up. It's not like you're here in a ripped T-shirt."

"I know," I said. He was right, it wasn't much of a before and after.

"I mean, the change should be on the inside, shouldn't it?"

"Yes," I said haltingly. "It should."

I frowned at the inelegant carpet on the convention-center floor, observing the effects of expensive scotch. I'd been pretty sure that the end-of-experiment picture idea was a good one, but now it seemed inane. Our apartment's elevator mirror hadn't shown me a radiant self-possessed personality beaming streams of inner beauty out upon the world—so who was it I was trying to snap a photo of? A stay-at-home mother who'd decided to quit sprucing herself up for her husband? A left-leaning writer struggling to adjust to the role of globetrotting corporate wife? A guilty aesthete who'd rejected beauty's materialism and bad politics yet remained a closet lover of Thierry Mugler and Christian Lacroix and who—in complete and utter secrecy—sometimes pulled the skin of her face back just to see what a facelift would do? Who was this person? A failure, a freak, and a sham?

"Forget it," I told John. "I don't need a picture."

"I can do it," he said.

"No," I said. "You're right. It doesn't make sense. Come on."

There was no making out in the cab on the way home; we just held hands and talked about John's projects and progress in the corporate hierarchy. I paid Mari, and John took the garbage out. Instead of spending a half hour in the bathroom taking off eye makeup, I waited for John to join me in the orange city glow that spread over our bed.

"Thanks for coming, babe," he said when he got in. "You looked nice."

"Mm."

"I'm sorry it's been so crazy. This Korea thing has just been . . . Well, I told you. The spring is going to be better. We should plan something."

"It might be hard to get the timing exactly right," I said, "but we could try for the cherry blossoms in Kyoto. While we have the chance."

"Hattie would love it. She loves flowers."

We were quiet a minute.

"How's your revision going?" John asked, referring to my novel, and reaching for my hand.

I told him, and more than I intended. I'd had to cut or rewrite the mountains of material I'd written in a tired or distracted haze during the early months of Hattie's life. I was hitting the deadlines I'd set for myself, but those efforts didn't seem to matter. A few days earlier, I'd picked up a book in a shop by someone I knew and skimmed through the first chapters. There was a clarity and directness to that storytelling voice that my own work lacked, and I knew it.

"Sometimes," I said, pressing the heels of my hands into my eye sockets, "I just wish I had different skills. I wish I found different things interesting and read different books, and used different words. Sometimes I just wish I was a *different writer*."

John said nothing to this. He didn't need to, because in his silence I heard it myself. Wanting to be a "different writer" sounded like wanting to be a person with a different dress size, less-wrinkled skin, better bone structure, more professional success, a better wardrobe, more time to work out, a cleaner house, and a more skillfully handled child. It sounded like wanting to be someone who embarked on a personal-improvement project that—one year in—felt absolutely like a resounding and permanent success.

Now I saw this pattern of longing for what it was: a habit born of fear. And with enough courage, it could change.

JANUARY ENDED, AND FEBRUARY PASSED. IT HAD NOW BEEN A FULL year since I purged my makeup bag and chopped my hair, but I put off my return to consumerdom, dithering. How would I handle the end of austerity? I thought about it every day. There was little risk that I'd go on a spree in De Beers, but I still felt safe, limited by the rules of my experiment. It had been such a struggle to move away from the black hole of consumer craving, and now that I was beyond it, I felt weightless. Being outside of desire was sublime, so why go back in?

I tested myself a few times. I went into Mannings drugstore, picked up a tube of mascara and a lipstick, put them back, picked them up again, purchased them, took them home, and let them roll to the back of my vanity table, unopened. I wandered into the knockoff handbag store on D'Aguilar Street and stood there noticing—but not identifying with—all the different identities a woman could project with her choice of straps, size of bag, and luxuriousness of materials. I didn't buy anything at that store, didn't even ask the salesperson to lift something off a shelf. I felt like I'd been to a distant land and returned, only to feel alien in my own home. The worst part of culture shock, say all the live-abroad guidebooks, is reentry.

One day I took Hattie on a grocery run to the Landmark. As I pushed her stroller briskly past the upscale stores, I spotted a white gown with purple crinoline on a dressmaker's dummy. It was adorned with a very long white veil. It was not a wedding gown, but it made me think of one, particularly the veil and train of the gown my friend Cate had worn. That was the first wedding I'd been in, a wedding that happened before any of my other friends were even dating the same person three weeks in a row. During the church rehearsal, the organ had roared, and every single person in the pews had leaped to his or her feet in honor of this holy prize, this miracle of beautiful, youthful fertility who was parading toward us in khaki shorts with a newspaper bouquet in her hands.

She's like a great big present, my inner Voice had said to me that day. *Girl as gift!* I was twenty-one then and didn't yet dream of marriage or children for myself. Rather cynically—with an anthropology degree in one hand and long list of hookups in the other—I saw my friend as so much of history had seen her: a fertile uterus in gift wrap. Now, years later, I saw the consequence, too. If a gift is what you were, then at some point, you were given away. Or you gave yourself away. And once that happened, there were no more proms or dates or dreams of happily ever after. No more magical boyfriends or waiting to be swept off your feet. No more "this is *my* day" events or ring shopping or gift showers or announcements that made all the older women in the room dab their eyes with vicarious delight. You were no longer the princess, no longer the bride, and no longer the beauty the whole world wanted.

At the beginning of my experiment, I'd felt this very thing. The sensation that I was already unwrapped—already used—infuriated me! How could this be? I was only thirty-two! I'd refused to believe it. In protest, I'd returned myself in a rage: chopping my hair, refusing to wear the gift wrap and ribbons, and denying that I was a treasure of youthful femininity.

Now, after my experiment's long year, that rage was gone. Instead, as I stood staring at the tulle and satin, I felt loss. It drifted over my shoulders like tossed petals. I looked down at my engagement ring, clouded with soap scum, and I wondered if Hattie would even remember the gift I once had been, as I had once gazed at my own mother.

Marching down the hardwood steps of my grandparents' house had been formal wedding portraits of my mother, my four aunts, and my grandmother. Each was framed in sterling, and each bride wore an ivory gown suited to her taste and fashion era. I'd spent long afternoons on those stairs as a child, falling in love with each separate instance of the matrimonial dream. Our own wedding photographer had not gotten a formal shot of me in my gown. I'd been a little annoyed by this in the weeks after our wedding, but thinking of it now brought me to tears. Yes, I'd probably spent too much time gazing at that parade of brides as a kid and not enough time reading about Curie, Goodall, Earhart, and Tubman. No, I didn't want Hattie to equate one day of loveliness with the pinnacle of female achievement. Still, it broke my heart to feel the brides—and my younger self with them—sweeping away into the distance, smelling of freesia and talcum, pulling long, spotless trains over the damp grass.

The dress and veil were on one side of the display window. My own reflection was on the other. I saw that there was no longer any chance of bringing the two together. Because of parenthood, and because of my age, my face, my waistline, my skin, and my experiment, I had grown. That lovely, old-fashioned silhouette for sale in the window was just too goddamned small.

In that moment, I listened for the Voice. If anyone could tell me what to do next, it would be her. But when I stilled my thoughts, I heard only the tinkle of piped-in classical music, and the clacking of heeled shoes as other shoppers passed.

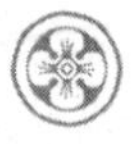

Snapshot: *Conversation with the Myth*

BOSTON, DECEMBER 2011

It's December now, the trees are bare, the holiday lights are everywhere, and it's the season of celebrating beloved myths. When I tell Hattie and Orson the old holiday stories, I play up the parts that matter to me: the birth of wisdom in a hay barn and the miracle of lamps that burn on belief. Whenever I can, I amp up the supervisory role of Mrs. Claus. Myths are vessels we pour the reality of our own lives into and make anew.

What I did during my experiment was reject a myth outright. It wasn't a considered choice, but a reflex that came from a place of deep hurt—how could the world be as meaningless or difficult as it truly is? It was also ultimately childish—if I couldn't have beauty as it was advertised, I wasn't going to settle for anything else. I was like the seven-year-old who tells all the little kids there's no such thing as the Tooth Fairy just to keep herself from crying over the loss.

Remaking a myth is a project of an entirely different order. It requires a realistic perception of culture's flexibility (not very), total mastery of the subject matter, compassion for the self as a believer, and a hard look at how much stake you lay in the story. Though I've tried, I haven't been able to pin down the exact moment the myth of youthful feminine perfection entered my life (a book of *Grimms' Fairy Tales*? A pack of pastel nightgowns? The *Solid Gold* dancers?).* I *do* know I started investing in the myth at a very early age, and although I wrestled with it a little in early adulthood ("Why should I wear nice clothes if I just want to take them off and act bad?"), I never had the heart to block out what the Voice of this myth whispered in my ear about the pinnacle of female beauty being a youngish me in a snowy-white wedding gown. When I hit close to that mark—on a warm August afternoon in a picturesque New England town—I figured I was in happily-ever-after territory and beyond reproach. I never dreamed that traveling overseas or becoming a parent would bring both this myth and its Voice screaming and snarking back into my life, meaner, nastier, and more self-loathing than she'd ever been before, possibly because, as she herself put it, *life feels so over already*. When a cherished myth runs up against its planned obsolescence, it isn't pretty.

I've heard some of my friends express similar sentiments—regardless of whether they have children or are married or have achieved any kind of professional success. One complained, "I feel like I went straight from thinking about which

---

* Tracking the development of this myth in your own life is an interesting exercise; for a prototype timeline, see my website, www.phoebebakerhyde.com.

miniskirt to wear to thinking about varicose veins. I was young and that was good, and then I was old and that was bad, and there was no in between." A stay-at-home mother cried, "I just want to feel like a woman again"—as if true, gratifying womanhood was something motherhood had taken away. When I expressed frustration at feeling weak and out of shape after pregnancy, a third reminded me darkly, "It's all downhill from here, baby." All four of us had excellent health, great educations, numerous professional prospects, money to pay for occasional child care, and accessible birth control. All of us were well under forty.

Survey Question

Have you ever felt that your real life doesn't match up with your own internal picture of success?

Always	6%
Often	24%
Sometimes	42%
Never	20%
I used to feel this way but got over it	6%

Although I wasn't conscious of it at the start, my experiment was not so much about silencing my inner Voice as getting her to grow up and get real. For much of my life, I'd let her weave my self-worth into the ancient tales of youthful beauty, and when these tales failed to instruct or guide, I thought I could just tune the Voice out and be rid of the myth like some ratty, old pink sweater. But the truth is that some parts of our psychic anatomy aren't our own. We inherit them like barrel chests and inward-turned pinkie toes, and we can't simply cut them out of ourselves without serious peril. So how do we reprogram that Voice to love and support the women we are instead of incessantly reminding us to step it up in the looks department because our beauty and youth are worth more to the planet than anything else?

Gently. Firmly. Compassionately. And, perhaps most important, a little bit at a time. I've become a fan of the term *generational advance.* I believe that every woman in a family line pushes the definition of womanhood a little further along and opens a few more doors to female worth. And as hard as it is, some of the old doors must be closed, too.

When John and I returned to the States, we went militant on pink princess paraphernalia—it was an imagination-killing virus that would not be seen in our house! I've since learned that complete royal banishment is impossible and foolhardy, but I've set limits and have never regretted the opportunity to ask Hattie what she thought a princess would do the day *after*

Survey Questions

How do you feel about princess, Barbie, Bratz, and other girly-girl products?

I don't like these products	35%
I have my reservations	39%
It's probably harmless	17%
Other opinion	4%
I love this stuff	4%

Do you believe in "happily ever after"?

Yes	58%
No	41%

her magical wedding, or to insist that any ballgown-wearing characters have skills, superpowers, and ambitions that reach well beyond looking good in a dress.*

In the long run, I suspect that the circumstances my kids see in real life will influence their decisions more than any enchanting stories they encounter. Hattie and Orson never think to question my working because it's what I've always done. They'll grow up eating at dinner tables where all kinds of lives and family choices are modeled, and gender is one in a range of identity points. I can't say for sure that John and I will ever achieve complete economic and labor parity in our marriage. But today Hattie and Orson have a mother who is neither at war with the mantle of womanhood nor stooped beneath it, but in daily conversation with her inner Voice about what it is, what it looks like, and what it can do.

JOHN WAFFLED, THIS YEAR, ABOUT WHETHER WE SHOULD GO TO HIS annual end-of-year party at all. The recession compelled his firm to give it up for a few years, and although it's back, it's far more subdued in the United States than in Hong Kong: simple cocktails and appetizers, an e-mail invitation, no grand theme. I suggested that I stay home and save the babysitting money for something else. John toyed with that idea for a few days

* There's been a recent groundswell of soul-searching about the princess ethos. Photographer Dina Goldstein evoked a massive love-hate response with her *Fallen Princesses* photographs online. A British organization called Pink Stinks demands less gendered choices in toys and clothes and calls on media to profile fewer footballers' wives and more women in science, health, and politics. Poetry slammer Katie Makkai cut through the fuzzy aura around the word *pretty* in a 2002 performance that went viral on YouTube. Finally, mom Cheryl Kilodavis wrote a children's book opening the whole princess ethos to boys.

and seemed to like it. But in the end he said, "I think I should be embracing this kind of stuff. We both should go."

On the night of the party, I put on the same black cocktail dress I now wear every year. Hattie knows about the infamous red dress in the back of my closet and wants me to wear it tonight because it is soft, bright, and fancy—halfway to costume.

"*When*, Mama, *when*?" she says, frustrated. "When are you gonna wear it?"

"One day," I tell her confidently. "Not tonight." I take out my engagement ring and slip it on. It's a lovely object and I value it tremendously, but it's full of cultural symbolism I'm still working out, and on most days I wear a simpler wedding band that matches John's.* Out of respect for my inner drama queen, though, I toss a tapestried shawl around my shoulders. It's an outfit.

"You look great," John says as we step out onto the street. I feel neither invisible nor over-the-top fabulous, just lucky to be going out with John to a party in our new city.

Overall, the firm's big holiday party is nice: there is food and drink, the conversations are short, the music is loud, and the dance floor crowded. After a while we take a handful of miniature cupcakes down to the level where a jazz quartet is playing, listen for a while, and then grab a taxi home.

We're quiet in the car, and at times like these I see evidence of John negotiating with his own myths of manhood.

---

* Diamond engagement rings became popular in the 1930s, the price of the ring roughly equaling the value of a woman's virginity. A broken engagement lessened a woman's chances for marriage and financial security, especially if she'd been deflowered by her fiancé. If things went wrong, she could always sell the ring and live off the proceeds. Before these rings, a man could be sued for breaking an engagement. Before that, brides-to-be were given thimbles, or their parents were given a cow. Before that, they might be tied up and delivered; a ring's most ancient symbolism is rope.

The ancient shapes are different for men—visually vaguer, perhaps, but more culturally rigid for their lack of being challenged much, yet. Questioning the stories of the self is hard work, sometimes scary, and usually slow. It doesn't have to be lonely, though. Committed couplehood is like two people holding hands and walking through a car wash. John didn't let go when I hit the big scrubber, and if it comes to that, I won't either.

At home, we sneak past our sleeping children, put on some favorite music, and dance. Sometimes we're together, sometimes apart—the elephant and the empress in her new clothes.

Burn Like the Sun at Midday

There is a special place in Hell for women who don't help other women.

—Madeline Albright, former US secretary of state and ambassador to the United Nations

Hong Kong, February and March 2008

I finally, formally, ended my experiment in March 2008, when a chronic time crunch pushed me back over the lip of consumerist rebellion and into the mall. John found a gap in his work schedule and—without any prompting, whining, demanding, or arm-twisting from me—took Hattie to Taiwan to visit relatives. It was a forty-eight-hour window of opportunity. I had loads of things I wanted to do with my time—reading, eating out—but my feet were sweaty and unsupported, my underpants were shredded, and for months my deflated breasts had been swimming in brassieres with underwires that dug into my skin. It was time.

Early on a Saturday morning, I headed out to Causeway Bay. If the elegant Landmark was the crowned head of retail in Hong Kong, then the Times Square mall complex was the beating heart. The nine-story shopping hub was positioned at the intersection of several major roads, surrounded by a maze-like pedestrian shopping district, and sat atop a subway artery that pumped shoppers directly into the basement. By three in the afternoon, crowd-control police would be needed, and there'd be a risk of being swept in the wrong direction by the hordes or getting slammed from behind by someone's overloaded stroller. Wary of these hazards, I arrived before ten, while the streets were still being swept up from the frenzy of the night before.

This trip began with promise. I did shoes first—comfortable sandals recommended by my podiatrist. I enjoyed trying on the colors and styles, found a pair I liked, and ordered them. Maybe I should get two pairs? Why do this more often than I had to? I got two.

Next I hit a British department store for the bras. I methodically destroyed the size 36 display rack, amassing a great pile of plastic hangers and cardboard packaging in the fitting room beside me. When I located the winning bra, I bought four in a range of useful, boring colors. Buoyed by this success, I waltzed into a shop for chic casualwear and tried on some jeans so awful in cut and fit I laughed out loud. I was feeling good. I was feeling strong. It was nearing noon when I spotted a crowded store known for reasonably priced designer copies. Why not go in and have a quick look before lunch?

Within ten minutes, my blood pressure was up, my heart was beating in time with the techno music, and I was moving from rack to rack scowling, pawing for my size, snarling at people who blocked the mirrors, and piling my arms with items I neither needed nor wanted. But they were being offered to me, and although none of them fit, or looked good, or delighted me in any way, I soldiered on, disbelieving my own dissatisfaction. Headache, dry mouth, and a bad case of mall-induced lower-back fatigue finally shut me down around three.

I hobbled away to a café to lick my wounds, carrying a plastic bag with a brown T-shirt in it I didn't even like very much. I bought an iced oolong tea and crumpled into a chair. What the hell had happened to me in there? Well, the music. The lighting. The prices. My own lack of a specific goal, whereas in the morning I'd had one. I took out my notebook, the nearly empty one in which I'd intended to record all my consumerist cravings all year, and wrote:

Shopping for things I need isn't leisure; it's a task, just like many others. And shopping for things I don't need yields buying things I don't need. (Plus a headache.)

I also wanted something to show for participating in all this unpleasantness.

I don't want to leave here empty-handed. But would it be so bad if I did?

I gulped down some headache medicine and thought about the new jeans I still didn't have. How could I do a better job buying those?

On the way home, I finally stopped into the new department store all my girlfriends had been raving about so many months ago. Like the designer-knockoff store, it was a danger zone of affordable delights. I tried on a lot of things, identified a few favorites, and then left. With nothing. The security guard was so suspicious of this madness, he checked the contents of my kiddie-stained backpack on my way out. How could anyone exit the store without at least one cheap, trendy garment? I did. I went home, had dinner, went to bed. The next morning, I went back there and plucked my favorites off the racks again. I checked to make sure I'd gotten the sizing correct and went up to the sales desk. I was in and out in about twenty minutes. By separating the delight of the costume box (day one) from the business of buying (day two) I'd avoided the quicksand of all-too-available desires. It felt like a success.

My End-of-Experiment Shopping Tally

Replacement Items

4 bras
10 underpants
2 bra-in tanks
1 pair of jeans
1 pair of pants
sunglasses with case
1 leather bag

New Items

2 yoga pants
3 shirts
2 pairs of orthotic sandals
1 pair of shorts

Total: $485 US

Whether I felt really terrific about spending the money at all was another issue. Back home, I collected my receipts, took them over to my empty jar, and looked at both. What I'd spent was not an overwhelming amount of money, or one that John would freak out over, especially since the most expensive items were shoes to remedy foot pain I'd been griping about for months. Still, it wasn't as if I'd spent the money on food, medicine, or charity. A year of self-reflection had highlighted many of my own needs in a positive and proactive way, but it had not erased the needy world that lay beyond: that Cameroonian schoolgirl I'd been inspired by or Blue-Flower Shirt, the homeless old woman who still sat near the back entrance of our building. I was still facing a crisis of conscience: how could I live with a self that needed new jeans once in a while, even when this trivial spending might mean so much more to another human being?

There's an old sawhorse about the Chinese character for crisis—it also means opportunity. I was still facing the same difficult intersection of female self-worth, history, money, and culture that I'd faced at the beginning of my experiment, but after these twelve-odd months, my perspective had changed. I'd seen that reliance on cosmetics was a symptom, not a sin; that inner and outer beauty were not have/don't have constructs; that modern partnerships needed something besides two opposed and inflexible roles; and that I had to remake the myths of femaleness, not reject them entirely. I knew that an either-or mentality would not help me deal with my empty jar, either; I had to honor altruism *and* self-interest. I wasn't sure how yet, but as a promise to those other women, I put my collection of shopping receipts in my empty jar as an IOU. Whether I'd done enough or too little was no longer the question. My future answer was doing more.

❧

THE WEEKEND THAT JOHN AND HATTIE WERE IN TAIWAN, I WENT out to sushi with Anne and Grace. It was an informal spot, but still, I'd just broken my fast and wanted to know: was I going to be a person who wore makeup and jewelry out with girlfriends, or one who did not?

As I showered and dressed, I thought of some fashion advice a friend had once given me, passed on from her grandmother. Turn away from the mirror, went the adage, and put on everything you want to wear. Then turn back to the mirror and remove the first thing you notice. It was a good rule for restraint, but I wondered if I could flip it around for an updated, postexperiment guideline: *Look in the mirror and appreciate everything already there: face, body, brain, health, love, kindness, intellect, strength. Add just one thing—for artistry, power, sex appeal, or fun. Now turn around and face the world.*

I liked this "one thing" idea, but that night I didn't follow it. I put on a favorite shirt and the new comfortable sandals, and then added a necklace and dangling gold earrings. I cracked open the mascara and lipstick I'd bought and put some of both on. I expected to be delighted with this adorned and enhanced self, but when I looked in the mirror, I was shocked by the difference between femaleness and femininity. Not necessarily enamored. There was a lot more recognizable womanhood in the mirror, but noticeably less of me. Something was also missing. I mugged for the camera. Yup, the big Vaseline smile was the finishing touch. It wasn't so bad, I convinced myself, plus I had to go.

My decorations lasted until I got in the taxi. I felt kittenish, overdone, and dishonest. I wiped off the lipstick and as much eye makeup as I could and stowed the earrings in my pocket. I left the necklace on, though, because it felt nicely cool against my collarbone. I went into the restaurant wearing, as it turned out, just one added thing.

A few days beforehand, Anne and I had gone out for pizza with the little girls, and I'd decided on the spot to tell her about my experiment. I'd been nervous and thick-tongued as I apologized for the omissions and explained why I'd not chimed in as often as I might have with the shopping talk.

Anne's reaction had been subdued and typically matter-of-fact. "You might have looked a bit grizzly now and then, but none of us are winning any pageants, are we?" She'd reached for a crust that Eva was flailing. "I really never noticed anything except the haircuts," she'd said, laughing, "and you told me all about those."

It was the best bubble-popping of my life. I'd guessed a year ago that Anne would be amused by the idea of my experiment. That she still was came as a tremendous relief. What had been emotionally wrenching for me could be a hoot for other women.

Since the subject was no longer off-limits, Anne, Grace, and I talked that night at sushi about how strange and eye-opening my experiment had been. I admitted how many questions it had raised, as opposed to providing answers. As we loitered at the counter, our conversation moving to other topics, I felt a total absence of appearance angst. I was just happy to be sitting at dinner with friends, my orthotically supported feet dangling off the stool, and nothing but soy sauce on my lips.

Anne and I walked home that night through the warm, familiar Hong Kong streets, passing its sights, signage, and people. Bankers in dark suits rushed up steps past the rainbow of vegetable vendors and drugstore advertisements, and a whiff of garlicky razor clams drifted out the open windows of a restaurant. There was a vast kaleidoscope of life ahead of me, inevitably filled with younger women flaunting better bone structure, cute shops hawking things I wanted but did not need, and those ongoing life challenges that had a habit of making themselves known through how I looked.

My experiment was over, but I knew my work wasn't done. Someday I'd tell Hattie: "You know, I went a year without makeup, jewelry, and new clothes once." If she asked me "Why?" or "What happened?" I didn't want to resort to saying "A lot of things," or "I don't really know." I wanted to have a story ready to tell—not an instructive fable or a magical fantasy—just a story about a real person living a real life. If I did it right, it wouldn't even need a happy ending with fireworks over a castle.

It would just need me.

Snapshot: *A Not-So-Big Reveal*

Boston, January 2012

Imagine a woman in the throes of getting ready to go out: jewels are strewn across the surface of the vanity, the lipstick and eyeliner are uncapped, smudged tissues are balled in corners, clothes are heaped on the bed, and the hairdryer is still warm. Everything has been used and tried. Everything has been hauled out and considered. Still, this woman is in her underwear. Her public face is half-finished and many of her decisions unmade. Her blood pressure is mounting as time ticks away—she has to wear something; she has to like it; it has to work. Above all, she has to recognize the necessity of imperfection: this thing is not solved, is not even solvable were she to spend her whole life figuring out what to wear! But enough already—she has to go. She has to get moving. Put something on the bottom. Put something on the top. Do something to the face; do something to the hair. Add the sparkle that lightens the heart. Find the shoes that soften the path, and go.

The woman above is the woman-I-was when I finished my experiment. Not fully pulled together, not closer to perfect, and not solved. This annoyed me, but I had to accept it. Shortly after I concluded my experiment, my life began a fast-forward no-brakes tumbling that is only now, almost four years later, beginning to slow. John was assigned to a long project in Tokyo, and Hattie and I went along so family life would be less disrupted. While we were there, we discovered I was pregnant with a second child, a fact that helped us make a decision to return to the States. I'd taken my experiment's notes to Japan, hoping to make something of them, but making an international move with a toddler, while pregnant, consumed most of my time and energy. This energy was not immediately forthcoming once the baby was born and I had to negotiate another new community. I did begin to read, however, and to listen to the voices of other women writers and thinkers who'd covered the same turf I found myself standing on. I kept my notes in a place where I could find them and kept an eye on myself as I faced the edifice of American culture.

Only a few days after our family returned to American soil, I recognized that I would never have hatched my experiment had I not been living abroad, an outsider in a foreign culture and foreign socioeconomic stratum. There's a real, marked difference between the freedom and power of American women and women elsewhere in the world, a difference that is reflected, perhaps, in a US tolerance for women wearing orthotic shoes, sweats, and no makeup, regardless of their social position. But what surprised me most upon my return was how ill-matched these new, real female lives were to an impossibly narrow standard of female beauty in the media, and to the crushing guilt so many of us carried because of the diva silhouette—guilt for not reaching it, guilt for trying so hard to and paying so much. In my first months at home, I kept thinking that the late-twentieth-century backlash against female advance had gone completely internal.

Today, when I talk with other women and men about my experiment and the frustration that impelled it, I notice two things.* First, very, very few men "get it" intuitively. Their response is usually to joke, "You tried not to worry about how you looked? I do that every day of my life! Har, har, har!" Although I don't think men are quite this callous about their appearance (they have to live in the world of power and sex, too), I think this response neatly demonstrates the invisible appearance handicapping that affects both sexes. Men feel a masculine requirement to mock the female Beauty Package, while women feel a requirement to produce and maintain it, even though both sides may be uncomfortable with its implications.

The second thing I notice is that women are very interested in the details. "What about your bikini line when you went swimming?" they ask, and "How did your husband feel?" I have tried to work these answers into the text, but the

---

* Three actually. In the company of aggressive naysayers, I've sometimes wished that I'd been more militant about my rules, forgoing every bit of jewelry, never depilating, and never falling off the wagon. I would have been more radical and more impressive. But impressiveness and impenetrability were never my aims. I had no book deal, no one watching over my shoulder, and only my own head to contend with. I did my experiment for myself and Hattie, and the wisdom I gained from my failures has proven far more useful in real life than any rhetorical fortress I might have built.

question that deserves its own space is "So what happened afterward? Did you go back to your old ways?"

The short answer is no. A lot of things have changed for good. My experiment's routine has become my daily routine: face splash, hairbrush, toothbrush, deodorant, and moisturizer. As the work-at-home parent of two small children, it takes about ten minutes of my day, which still sometimes feels like more than I can afford. Free time is still a luxury for me, but sleep no longer is. I count my eight-hour average up there with food, water, and shelter. As far as body-hair maintenance, I've settled on a policy of seasonal reduction rather than constant removal. Learning more about what's in makeup has caused me to chuck all my chemically based foundations, tanners, bronzers, whiteners, and wrinkle correctors, as well as phase out pthalates, parabens, hormone disrupters, and petroleum. I have slapped a little Band-Aid over an occasional big zit, but when blemishes, undereye circles, eczema, sallow skin, or bloodshot eyes become the norm, I take the time to investigate an underlying health problem.

What hasn't changed is a desire to look my best when those looks are important, and a delight in getting dressed up from time to time. When I go to see friends or meet with colleagues, I think about my clothes and look in the full-length mirror. But I do so with an eye that discriminates between looking my best and looking like a gift-wrapped set of reproductive organs. Women have done end runs around anatomy before with jogging bras, tampons, PMS medications, and the Pill, and I see no reason we can't manage the magnet of sexual attraction to serve our best everyday interests as well. For those once-or-twice-a-year traditional social events, I do use a few of the old-school enhancements: jewelry, mascara and lip tint, low-heeled shoes. I might fool with my hair and try on a few different outfits. When Hattie watches me from her post on the toilet seat, I tell her that this is an event for which her Mama and Baba need to be Miz Lovely McDovely and Mr. Handsome Dansome. If she and Orson attend, they get to be Pretty McDitty and Cutie Patootie. She gets it, I think: there is artifice involved, and some cultural expectation, but these can be fun.

Our downfall—Hattie and me—is hair. She wants hers long; I want it brushed. She wants mine long; I've embraced my short hair now, but prefer it the shade it was before pregnancy darkened it. I spritz mine with a homemade mix of lemon and peroxide sometimes to lighten it up. When we remember, Hattie and I cooperate to braid or ponytail her hair before school.

"You can always just cut it off," I tell her, brushing. "It would be a lot easier."

"I know," she says. "Maybe in the summer."

The truth is that I love her straight, satiny dark hair; love my lighter, wavier own; and love that they are so different. It took me five years to accept it, but I already know I'm not the only role model she'll ever look up to, or need. For this reason, I'm grateful for all my girlfriends who make appearance choices different from mine, for all the parents who don't choke on pink, and for all the women out there making life work in their designer clothes, stilettos, or three-inch manicures. I have come to see that what I really care about is not the nuances of appearance as much as the messages they send about deeper human challenges we all face.

I used to feel that work on the self and work on the world were miles apart. Today, I see these two needs as two sides of the same puzzle, with my own capacity for compassion and generosity completing the picture. It was my survey respondents who best helped me realize that if I wanted to share with others, I had to feel I had enough, and had to value my assets and be valued in turn. By confronting my own problems—by not covering them up or prettifying them—I feel empowered to go out to a much more troubled world, one that too often has the face of female pain and suffering.

Since the end of my experiment I've finally begun to pay a portion of my beauty wealth forward. My donations were very small—but a start. Through Po Leung Kuk, a social services organization in Hong Kong, I donated to mental health support systems for recent Mainland immigrants, particularly women and families in the "City of Sadness." I also contacted a home for the elderly in the neighborhood where we'd lived. They had no information about Blue-Flower Shirt, but hopefully my donation will help prevent another's similar fate. I gave to UNFPA, the UN-sponsored leader in global maternal-fetal health initiatives, and through Kiva.org I invested in women's entrepreneurial projects around the world. Finally, I kept my promise to that barefoot Cameroonian schoolgirl by giving to Strategic Humanitarian Services in Cameroon, one of the many school-building charities hard at work there. What attracted me to SHUMAS was the wide scale of their work and the strong Cameroonian project leadership. The clincher, however, was a note on their website about the problem of "jiggers." Barefoot kids learning on dirt floors often have trouble with foot parasites. New schools will help, but so would flip-flops. Beauty is a lens we adjust for ourselves; my experiment helped me redefine the term *must-have shoes.*

Survey Questions

Percentage of female respondents who give regularly to a cause, institution, political group, or organization that promotes their values or beliefs: 66%

Top-five issues that respondents empathize with and which cause them to help others:

- getting educated or providing school
- women's health
- intellectual, political, or religious freedom
- discrimination
- domestic or sexual violence

My search for inner beauty—or whatever I thought I meant by it—has far outlasted my experiment and seeped into every corner of my life. Although it's still easy to wish for otherness, it's better, if harder, to become the parent and partner I truly am, and to find beauty in the voice I already have.

Today, if I wake up right now to what is happening around me moment by moment—the lemon-yellow sun on a fence across the street, the whir of the heater at my ankles as I work—I feel this book closing very gently, with a whisper. Part of me resists. Our era loves a makeover and a set of makeover shots—a big reveal. But we all know by now that personal change isn't so easy, doesn't come cheap or overnight, and never replaces flaws with perfection.

Still, change does happen, and must happen as years pass. Beauty, life, and growth all depend on change. Every day we are alive is an "after" shot, as well as a "before." In the introduction to this book, I said I could lay claim to feeling beautiful, and for this I credit the Koine Greeks' concept of beauty. Their word for it was *horaios*: to be of one's hour, a thing perfectly expressing the characteristics of its age. It could be the new bud or the blown rose. It could be a woman whose youth and promise are breathtaking, or a woman whose health and wisdom give grace to her age. It could be a woman like me—a woman at the midpoint of life, burning like the sun at midday.

A FINAL SNAPSHOT. IT IS 7:45 A.M., TWENTY DEGREES, AND JOHN, Hattie, Orson, and I are tumbling out the door on our way to work and school.

In his fedora and dark suit, John looks as if he stepped out of the 1950s, but this is a sly misrepresentation. He got Orson dressed this morning and supervised both kids in toothbrushing and lunch-box packing. He has agreed to rearrange some work calls so he can be home tonight while I get out to a reading, and he's anticipating tryouts for a local orchestra next month. If John is "the man," the man has subtly and fundamentally changed.

I am, at the moment, deep in my role as reluctant family drill sergeant, but I take it more lightly in my fur-edged czarina coat. Underneath I have on my holey jeans and lucky engineered socks.

"Keys, Mama," Hattie reminds me with precise competence. She stands in the doorway in her snow boots, her glitter slippers tucked wisely in her backpack. She is quiet, possibly visualizing the number line, or the clay figurine she has been working on, or the fish sticks she will eat at lunch. As she holds the door, Orson blows past her in an unzipped jacket and a tiger hat. He leaps into the morning, biting at it.

You can see it best in winter—how we bundle ourselves daily in layer after layer of artistry and identity and lug along with us, like so many lunch boxes and backpacks, some daily baggage about how we will be treated and how the day will go.

But when I breathe in the first dagger of cold air, I feel how close I am to the raw beauty of this morning itself. The arctic temperature stings my face. There are wet-looking patches of ice on the uphill; Orson dashes across as Hattie clings to my arm, and we go more cautiously together under the trees. John suddenly turns, presses his warm, chapped lips to mine for a half second, and bounds across traffic for the train. My heart skips up as he goes—for fear, delight, and panic at the passing of time and the unpredictable movement of big vehicles and small children, for awe of the real thing that is me, paused on a street corner shivering with joy.

This is it, whispers the Voice. *Don't miss it.*

About the Survey

THE BEAUTY EXPERIMENT WOMEN'S SURVEY was a forty-two-question assay of female attitudes toward beauty and was accompanied by a ten-question Men's Survey. Both were posted on my website on June 30, 2010, and administered, tallied, and cross-tabulated by SurveyGizmo, a well-known third-party survey provider. Invitations to complete my surveys were issued through my own e-mail and Facebook networks and later publicized in venues I selected: on Facebook ads and in online chat rooms of magazines. (I was able to post in *Bust, Cosmo, FHM, Good Housekeeping, GQ, Marie Claire,* and *More.*) Of the thousands who likely viewed my posts and ads, only a few hundred self-selected to respond. These individuals did not get paid and were kept geographically and electronically anonymous.

By January 24, 2011, I had 470 complete responses from women and 112 from men. (While someone pointed out that I can't verify that everyone who took my women's survey was a woman, I can share that the four men who erroneously started to take the women's survey wrote funny frustrated things in the comment boxes and gave up.) It is important to note that both surveys are emphatically "snowball" surveys, meaning my results were intended not for academic scrutiny but for lighthearted discussion, like a reader poll, or magazine quiz. Sample size and demographic distribution were not controlled for, a shortcoming that is probably reflected in the fact that the majority of respondents reported living in households with incomes of more than fifty thousand dollars a year. In this book, results have been rounded to the nearest whole number, and not every question has been included for reasons of space and relevance. The percentages I cite are also descriptive statistics, representative *only of my survey takers* and not of any larger group, such as women, or American women, or even women between the ages of thirty and thirty-nine. When I speak of women at large in the text, I am doing so as an essayist and cultural critic, not as a social scientist.

In writing my questions and answers, I did consult with a sociologist and other professional data gatherers, all of whom exhorted me to limit the scope of my survey and generalize my language to remove bias. While doing this made my survey hideously more boring to take, I followed orders and provided fill-in text boxes when I thought respondents might feel pushed into corners. Despite these measures, I still ran afoul of many. To them I apologize for being a writer, not a researcher, and warmly invite them to post on my website, sharing any positions I failed to imagine. When I scroll through the surveys today, I am more than anything humbled by my respondents' generosity toward my project, and I remain forever grateful for their proof of beauty's alluring paradoxes.

Notes

Chapter 1: The Red Dress

5 **I'd thought I could negotiate:** Measurements of the average Chinese woman come from Alvanon, the Global Size and Fit Expert, "Alvanon Releases Most Extensive Chinese Body Measurement Survey," August 12, 2008, www.alvanon.com/news/CHINASCAN.pdf.

18 **One supplement aimed at preventing an iodine deficiency:** Nicholas D. Kristof and Sheryl WuDunn, *Half the Sky: Turning Oppression into Opportunity for Women Worldwide* (New York: Alfred A. Knopf, 2009), 173.

18 **Hong Kong itself has a legendary wealth differential:** Natalie Wong, "More Fall into Poverty Trap," *Standard,* October 4, 2010, www.thestandard.com.hk/news_detail.asp?pp_cat=30&art_id=103468&sid=29803867&con_type=1.

20 **I did discover that the cost:** IRIN Humanitarian News and Analysis, "Zimbabwe: Soaring Tuition Fees Deprive Youth of Education," February 28, 2007, www.irinnews.org/InDepthMain.aspx?InDepthId=28&ReportId=70041&Country=Yes.

Chapter 3: The Hair Questions

40 **an average of seven months:** Mohit Joshi, "British Women Spend Hair Raising £27,722 on Haircare!" *TopNews*, January 23, 2008, http://www.topnews.in/health/british-women-spend-hair-raising-27-722-haircare-2731a.

44 **an age-old human quirk:** Mimi Spencer, "Why Can't We Just Let Our Hair Down?" *Guardian*, January 22, 2003, www.guardian.co.uk/world/2003/jan/23/gender.uk.

Chapter 4: Two Half-Moons of Peach Paste

51 **the legal minimum wage for foreign domestic workers:** Immigration Department HKSAR, *Foreign Domestic Helpers FAQ's*, www.immd.gov.hk/eht/faq_fdh.htm#4 (accessed July 30, 2012); Kent Ewing, "Soon in Hong Kong: Invasion of the Amahs," *Asia Times*, August 4, 2011, www.atimes.com/atimes/china/mh04ad01.html.

52 **Seventy-two consecutive hours of lost sleep:** William C. Dement, MD, PhD, and Christopher Vaughn, *The Promise of Sleep: A Pioneer in Sleep Medicine Explores the Vital Connection Between Health, Happiness, and a Good Night's Sleep* (New York: Delacorte, 1999), 63, 219, 224, 231, 262, 265, 398.

60 **excessive grooming is a known anxiety reliever:** Renee Montagne interview with Dr. Barbara Natterson Horowitz, author of *Zoobiquity: What Animals Can Teach Us About Health and the Science of Healing*, NPR on Facebook, June 12, 2012.

61 ***Today Show* anchors Kathy Gifford and Hoda Kotbe:** Vida Rao, "KLG, Hoda Dare to Bare (Their Faces)," *Today Show* at MSNBC, May 13, 2010, http://today.msnbc.msn.com/id/37130121.

62 **Particularly at risk of being affected:** Thirteen out of twenty teen girls tested by the watchdog organization Environmental Working Group had hormone-disrupting chemicals in their blood, including phthalates, triclosan, parabens, and musks. Rebecca Sutton, PhD, "Adolescent Exposures to Cosmetic Chemicals of Concern," September 2008, www.ewg.org/reports/teens.

Chapter 5: The Day I Covered the Mirrors

82 **"Women watch themselves":** John Berger, *Ways of Seeing* (London: BBC and Penguin Books, 1972), 47.

83 **women and girls are fated:** Kate Fox, "Mirror, Mirror: A Summary of Findings on Body Image," Social Issues Research Centre, 1997, www.sirc.org/publik/mirror.html.

84 **women check their faces in the mirror:** This survey of two thousand people was commissioned by Transformulas International, a British cosmeceutical company. While the average number of times these women looked in the mirror was thirty-four, in individual cases the number could be much higher. "British Women Look in the Mirror 71 Times a Day," *Marie Claire,* November 5, 2007, www.marieclaire.co.uk/news/beauty/160829/british-women-look-in-mirror-71-times-a-day.html.

Chapter 6: Itsy Bitsy Teeny-Weeny Fertility Advertisement

89 **From zaftig Marilyn to skinny Kate Moss:** For a wonderfully in-depth analysis of the biology behind human appreciation for physical beauty, see Nancy Etcoff, *Survival of the*

Prettiest: The Science of Beauty (New York: Anchor Books, 2000), 190–194.

101 **Any woman of any race in the world:** Ibid., 57, 138.

101 **most brides in traditional cultures:** Ibid., 57.

Chapter 7: The Professionals

113 **Good looks have been proven to protect individuals:** Nancy Etcoff, *Survival of the Prettiest: The Science of Beauty* (New York: Anchor Books, 2000), 25, 44–52.

117 **The female leaders were all given three-quarter-length portraits:** Platon, "Portraits of Power," *New Yorker,* December 7, 2009, 51–77, www.newyorker.com/online/multimedia/2009/12/07/091207_audioslideshow_platon. The photographs can be viewed online, but are cropped differently.

118 **projected to grow by five trillion dollars in the next five years:** Doug Anderson, "Below the Topline: Women's Growing Economic Power," Nielsen Consulting Group, October 6, 2009, http://blog.nielsen.com/nielsenwire/global/below-the-topline-womens-growing-economic-power/.

118 **According to the Bureau of Labor Statistics:** Bureau of Labor Statistics, "Personal Care Activities Done by Men and Women in 2009," American Time Use Survey, www.bls.gov/tus/current/personal.htm#a1 (accessed February 26, 2012).

118 **A great example of this grooming differential:** Michel Luo, "Top Salary in McCain Camp? Palin's Makeup Stylist," *New York Times,* October 24, 2008, http://thecaucus.blogs.nytimes.com/2008/10/24/palins-makeup-stylist-fetches-highest-salary-in-2-week-period/.

Chapter 8: Pretty Mind

125 **this domestic valley of shadow:** Sylvia Plath, *Ariel* (1965; reprint, New York: Harper Perennial, 1999); for the wickedly funny version, see contemporary novelist Jill Kargman's *Momzillas* (New York: Broadway Books, 2007).

128 **this personal growth/self-help book:** Karen Maezen Miller, *Momma Zen: Walking the Crooked Path of Motherhood* (Boston: Trumpeter, 2007).

131 **"to live deliberately":** Henry D. Thoreau, *Walden and Resistance to Civil Government,* 2nd ed. (New York: W. W. Norton, 1992), 60.

Chapter 9: A Language Every Body Speaks

142 **studies have recently found a higher density of nerve endings:** Melinda Wenner, "Women's Better Sense of Touch Explained," *Scientific American,* April 30, 2010, www.scientificamerican.com/article.cfm?id=womens-better-sense-of-touch-explained.

144 **There have been several fashion experimenters:** Martin's project no longer has a website, but Zittel's project can be found at www.zittel.org/work.php, and Matheiken's project can be found at https://theuniformproject.com. To read about all three, see Rob Walker, "This Year's Model," *New York Times Magazine,* July 9, 2009, www.nytimes.com/2009/07/12/magazine/12fob-consumed-t.html?_r=2&ref=magazine.

158 **two-week runway-to-sales rack turnaround:** Eric Wilson, "Before Models Can Turn Around, Knockoffs Fly," *New York Times,* September 4, 2007, www.nytimes.com/2007/09/04/us/04fashion.html?pagewanted=all.

158 **an average 300 percent retail markup:** Kentin Waits, "Cheat Sheet: Retail Markup on Common Items," *Wisebread*, December 15, 2010, www.wisebread.com/cheat-sheet-retail-markup-on-common-items.

158 **a legion of people with box cutters standing by:** Jim Dwyer, "A Clothing Clearance Where More than Just the Prices Have Been Slashed," *New York Times*, January 5, 2010, www.nytimes.com/2010/01/06/nyregion/06about.html.

158 **sixty tons per day:** Goodwill Facts, "Reduce, Reuse, Recycle," *Amazing Goodwill*, www.amazinggoodwill.com/categories/6-reducereuserecycle/documents/7-reduce-reuse-recycle (accessed February 26, 2012). To see what thirty tons of discarded clothing looks like, see photos of Christian Boltanski's *No Man's Land* at the Park Avenue Armory in 2010. This pile was borrowed from a secondhand clothes dealer who moves twice this amount daily. "Clothes Horse: Christian Boltanski at the Park Avenue Armory in NYC," C-monster.net, May 14, 2010, http://c-monster.net/blog1/2010/05/14/christian-boltanski/.

158 **garments made out of questionable fabrics and sewn in less-than-ideal conditions:** For a good discussion of cotton production, polyester, and what's really "green" in textiles, see Yvonne Zipp, "Before You Buy Those Organic Blue Jeans . . . ," *Christian Science Monitor*, September 29, 2008, www.csmonitor.com/Environment/Living-Green/2008/0929/before-you-buy-those-organic-bluejeans.

Chapter 10: The Empty Jar

175 **one of the 90 percent of women who felt financially insecure:** Suze Orman, *Women and Money: Owning the*

Power to Control Your Destiny (New York: Speigel and Grau, 2007), 8.

175 **younger women ages twenty-five to thirty-four:** Hannah Seligson, "The Shopaholic Myth," *Slate.com,* November 10, 2010, www.slate.com/id/2274416/.

176 **asked working mothers how they relieved stress:** Survey commissioned for Cathy L. Greenberg and Barret S. Avigdor, *What Happy Working Mothers Know* (Hoboken, NJ: Wiley and Sons, 2009).

176 **a culturally sanctioned habit of retail therapy:** Lawrence Haddad, John Hoddinott, and Harold Alderman, eds., *Intrahousehold Resource Allocation in Developing Countries* (published for the International Food Policy Research Institute by Johns Hopkins University, 1997), www.ifpri.org/publication/intrahousehold-resource-allocation-developing-countries-0.

176 **If the beauty industry has an annual revenue of $10 billion:** "Cosmetics, Beauty Supply, and Perfume Retail Industry Description," *Hoover's,* www.hoovers.com/industry/cosmetics-beauty-supply-perfume-retail/1528-1.html (accessed February 26, 2012).

Chapter 11: Outgrowing the Gown

200 **groundswell of soul-searching about the princess ethos:** The queen of the antiprincess movement is Peggy Orenstein, who wrote the *Cinderella Ate My Daughter: Dispatches from the Front Lines of the New Girlie-Girl Culture* (New York: HarperCollins, 2010). To see Goldstein's princess shots, go to www.fallenprincesses.net. For Pink Stinks, see www.pinkstinks.co.uk/. For Katie Makkai's poetry slam, see www.youtube.com/watch?v=M6wJl37N9C0&feature=email.

For Cheryl Kilodavis, see www.myprincessboy.com/index.asp.

201 **a simpler wedding band:** For a pointed history of the engagement ring, see Meghan O'Rourke, "Diamonds Are a Girl's Worst Friend: The Trouble with Engagement Rings," *Slate.com*, June 11, 2011, http://www.slate.com/articles/news_and_politics/weddings/2007/06/diamonds_are_a_girls_worst_friend.html.

Readings

IN ADDITION TO THOSE CITED IN MY NOTES, these books inspired and informed, and helped me put my story in historical, cultural, and philosophic context:

Anger: Wisdom for Cooling the Flames by Thich Nhat Hanh

The Beauty Bias: The Injustice of Appearance in Life and Law by Deborah L. Rhode

The Beauty Myth: How Images of Beauty Are Used Against Women by Naomi Wolf

Bring Me the Rhinoceros, and Other Zen Koans to Bring You Joy by John Tarrant

Creating a Life: Professional Women and the Quest for Children by Sylvia Ann Hewitt

The Feminine Mystique by Betty Friedan

Flux: Women on Sex, Work, Love, Kids, and Life in a Half-Changed World by Peggy Orenstein

Going Grey: What I Learned About Beauty, Sex, Work, Motherhood, Authenticity, and Everything Else That Really Matters by Anne Kreamer

A Haunted House, and Other Short Stories and *To The Lighthouse* by Virginia Woolf

I Am Nujood, Age 10 and Divorced by Nujood Ali with Delphine Minoui

I Feel Bad About My Neck, and Other Thoughts on Being a Woman by Nora Ephron

In the Company of Women: Turning Workplace Conflict into Powerful Alliances by Pat Heim, Susan Murphy, and Susan K. Golant

The Invisible Dragon: Essays on Beauty by Dave Hickey

Maidenhome by Ding Xiaoqui

A Proper Marriage by Doris Lessing

Speak, Memory by Vladimir Nabokov

This Is Not How I Thought It Would Be by Kristin Maschka

Woman: An Intimate Geography by Natalie Angier

Women by Annie Leibovitz, with an introduction by Susan Sontag

Acknowledgments

FOR WHATEVER BEAUTY THIS BOOK POSSESSES, I owe great thanks to Sorche Fairbank, Katie McHugh, and all at Da Capo for believing in it and bringing it to print. Writers/editrixes Ariane Conrad, Andrea Troyer, and Lisa Turvey enriched the manuscript greatly with their intelligence and sensitivity; Rahna Reiko Rizzuto saw me through a dark hour of revision, Suzie Roth Design produced the dazzling Beauty Experiment website, and Lucinda Brown and Professor Robin Leitner of the University of Pennsylvania were instrumental in the development of the Beauty Experiment Surveys. A 572-gun salute to each of the family members, friends, fellow parents, former classmates, and complete strangers who took the survey and then generally spread it around. Special commendation to all family members, Emilie Boggis, Flannery Burke, Caitlin Boyle, Hartford Gongaware, and Heidi Osborne for key dispersals.

To all those in my Hong Kong tribe who kept me sane and looking forward to Fridays and meet-ups in the park, I raise a strong, properly prepared cup of tea with milk and sugar. The experience of living abroad was a high mark against which I will measure the rest of my life. To my friends in Chatham, a heartfelt thanks for your encouragement and for providing a home we still miss daily. For wrangling my young children with gentleness and great care during the writing of this book, I bow to M-C. K., J. K., and the staff of the Tiny World. I am indebted to Michelle Latiolais for being a literary and personal mentor of unparalleled wisdom for this and many other projects, and I am grateful to the MFA program at the University of California at Irvine for academic, financial, and creative support. To those many dear longtime friends who appear in this book and/or have been cheering me on for decades, this is just one of a lifetime of thank-yous.

For their patience and unquestioning support of every kind, I have to thank the entire Hyde and Liang families, particularly my parents, who taught me that the best way to deal with a terrifying eyeball in the grass is to cut it open with a knife. John, Hattie, and Orson I can never thank enough except by doing this work, because it is the best I can do.